The Diet Survivor's Handbook

60 Lessons in Eating, Acceptance and Self-Care

Judith Matz and Ellen Frankel

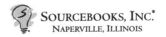

SOURCEBOOKS, INC.
NAPERVILLE, ILLINOIS

Published by Sourcebooks, Inc.
P.O. Box 4410, Naperville, Illinois 60567-4410
(630) 961-3900
Fax: (630) 961-2168
www.sourcebooks.com

Library of Congress Cataloging-in-Publication Data

Matz, Judith
  The diet survivor's handbook : 60 lessons in eating, acceptance, and self-care / Judith Matz and Ellen Frankel.
      p. cm.
  1. Reducing diets--Psychological aspects. 2. Weight loss--Psychological aspects--Popular works. 3. Food habits--Psychological aspects--Popular works. I. Frankel, Ellen. II. Title.

RM222.2.M3793 2006
613.2'5--dc22

2005025121

Printed and bound in the United States of America
POD 10 9 8 7 6 5 4 3 2

We dedicate this book to diet survivors:
may you find courage and inspiration in
these pages.

Contents

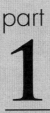

part

1

Becoming a
DIET SURVIVOR

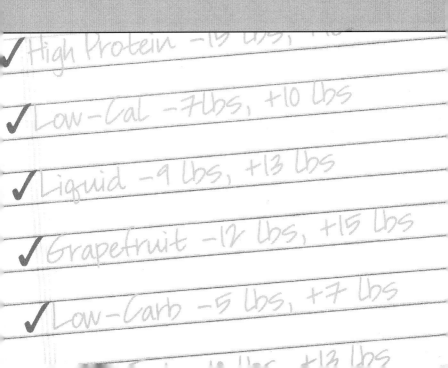

✓ High Protein −19 lbs, +10 lbs

✓ Low-Cal −7 lbs, +10 lbs

✓ Liquid −9 lbs, +13 lbs

✓ Grapefruit −12 lbs, +15 lbs

✓ Low-Carb −5 lbs, +7 lbs

−19 lbs, +13 lbs

It's NOT Your Fault

"I have not failed.
I've just found 10,000 ways that won't work."
—*Thomas Edison*

How many books have you opened searching for the ultimate solution for weight loss? How many times have you promised yourself that a new diet would be *the* diet, the one-that-would-really-work diet, the one-that-would-change-your-life diet? How many times were your hopes lifted as the pounds dropped, only to be dashed as the weight ultimately returned? The allure of dieting is everywhere, along with the promise that once you become thinner through dieting, everything—absolutely everything—will change for the better. So you spend a good portion of your days, weeks, months, and years waiting to lose weight so that your life can truly begin. As a diet survivor, the life you have always wanted to live can begin *today.*

In 2000, the number of Americans dieting to lose weight totaled nearly 116 million people, representing 55 percent of the adult population. Yet approximately 95 to 98 percent of all dieters who lose weight will ultimately regain the lost pounds, often leading to higher than pre-diet weights. The diet industry, which takes in approximately $50 billion a year, has a failure rate unthinkable in any other consumer area. Can you imagine a doctor prescribing a medication that offered a 2 percent chance of curing you? And when your illness persisted, would you blame yourself? But because of the popular belief that dieting will make you thin, people try one weight loss method after another. In the process, they become yo-yo dieters caught in a vicious cycle, blaming themselves for their diet failures.

For most, the thought of giving up dieting is equivalent with the notion of giving up on themselves. It means forgoing thinness and the promises of health, happiness, and success equated with this cultural ideal. However, dieting is inherently dangerous. Diets leave a trail of devastating physical and emotional consequences in their wake. Anyone who can stop this cycle is a diet survivor!

The fact that you are reading these pages speaks to the part of you that has been wondering, considering, and assessing the merit of diets—the part of you that is sick and tired of riding the diet roller coaster and measuring your life by the number on a scale. *If you have been on more than one diet, lost and regained the weight, and are becoming aware that the failure is not your fault, you are a diet survivor.*

The use of the term *survivor* is commonly used in reference to a person who is faced with dire circumstances and obstacles who, nonetheless, triumphs. Calling a person who is able to give up dieting a survivor gives credence both to the damage caused by diets and to the empowerment that results when people move from a diet mentality to a normal relationship with food. The term *diet survivor* encourages people to get off the diet roller coaster and get on the non-diet bandwagon of living fully and joyfully in one's body through the life-affirming action of feeding oneself based on internal cues of hunger and satiety.

What do diet survivors have in common? Every survivor knows how to lose weight. They know how to count calories, fat grams, carbohydrates, or whatever is in vogue for the moment. They know the wonderful feeling that comes from shedding pounds and receiving compliments from friends, family, and coworkers. They know the incredible control and pride they feel when they pass up their favorite dessert. They also know the relief of breaking through the diet restraints when they finally give in to their cravings, and they know all too well the feelings of being out of control that accompany a binge. They know the harshness of the internal voice telling them they are weak and disgusting. And they know the fear that they will never get back on track. They know the shame of regaining the lost weight and the pain when friends, family, and coworkers fall silent.

But what diet survivors also have in common is the fact that they are in the process of making a transformation. Rather than remaining in a damaging downward spiral, they embark on a journey toward physical and psychological well-being. They are reaching the conclusion that they cannot tolerate one more diet. They are saying "no" to deprivation and "no" to the overeating that inevitably follows. They are no longer willing to sacrifice their health and happiness to lose weight. They are tired of feeling depleted by their preoccupation with food and weight and of waiting for a number on the scale to give them permission to start living.

But saying "no" is not enough. In order to make significant changes, diet survivors must develop and embrace positive attitudes and behaviors that lead to a satisfying relationship with food, their bodies, and themselves. Can you imagine what it would be like to wake up and feel as if the possibilities of your life were spread before you? What if your days were no longer defined as good or bad based on weight and you no longer constricted yourself to diets?

In our culture, it's hard to imagine having a life you feel entitled to live fully and freely regardless of weight. We have been taught that rewards are offered to those who conform to the celebrated ideal of thin, and we are encouraged to pursue this body type at all costs.

If you are like most dieters, you want to lose weight more than anything. We know how hard you have tried. You've dieted to lose weight more than once, attempting different kinds of weight loss programs or food plans. There is a good chance that others have encouraged you to pursue your weight loss goals. With each diet, you probably lost some weight. This always feels wonderful because it seems like you are getting your eating under control. Losing weight also means that you receive compliments, fit into smaller sizes, and feel a boost of confidence.

With such benefits, it's interesting that virtually all dieters regain the weight. You have to wonder why this is happening when you, and other dieters like you, want so desperately to be thin and are so pleased with the weight loss. Has anyone ever told you that it is not your fault that the pounds have returned? Let us tell you this now. *It is not your fault.* The flaw is in the diet itself. For all but a very small number of dieters the lost weight is regained, often leading to higher weights than before the diet. When this happens, you are likely to feel some or all of the following:

- I am weak; a stronger person could have kept the weight off.
- I am bad; a good person would have stayed on the diet and become thin.
- I am lazy; I cannot be counted on to succeed.
- I feel helpless; I don't know what to do to lose weight and make my body acceptable.
- I feel shame; I'm embarrassed that I failed and am disgusted with my appearance.

You will also find yourself feeling out of control with food when you break through the restraints of your diet.

Eating more food than you need and eating foods that you consider to be bad for you are natural responses to the deprivation induced by dieting.

What We Know

The reason we can predict these feelings and behaviors is because dieting creates a scenario with predictable results. Later, we will explain why that scenario occurs. For now, we want to emphasize that the failure of diets and the accompanying feelings are *normal* reactions to the cycle of dieting. Regardless of why you first started dieting, the types of diets tried, or even the number of pounds lost and regained, you share certain experiences as a result of these attempts.

Going on a diet is a response to negative feelings or thoughts about yourself. "I'm too fat," "I'm unhealthy," "My stomach sticks out," or "I am out of control with food" are typical comments that might motivate you to lose weight. When you begin your diet, you feel a great sense of hopefulness. "This time," you tell yourself, "I am going to stick to the diet, lose weight, and feel so much better." For a time, you adhere to the rules of your food plan. This sense of control makes you feel good, especially when you begin to lose weight and receive compliments.

Eventually, however, you break the restraints of your diet. Perhaps you are at a party and the dessert looks too good to pass up, or a particularly stressful day causes you to head to the refrigerator. When you go off your diet, you feel upset and criticize yourself for losing control. At the same time, you find it hard to stop eating. After all, you've already broken the rules. You figure you might as well eat whatever you want now because in the near future you will need to go back on the same diet or try a new one. The weight you lost returns. Instead of receiving compliments, there is silence from the people in your life. This combination of events causes you to feel bad about yourself and your behavior. These negative feelings will lead you to the next diet, perpetuating the cycle of dieting and overeating.

When a pattern occurs in such a predictable way, *it can no longer be considered a personal failure.* Rather, the fact that certain feelings, behaviors, and consequences occur frequently and consistently for people in a particular situation means that the problem lies outside of the individual, regardless of his or her own unique set of circumstances. *You haven't failed diets; diets have failed you.*

Although you have heard the phrase "diets don't work," you may believe that you will be one of the lucky few who can successfully control what you eat. You may think that if only you are more determined, you will keep the pounds off. If only you can find the diet that *really* works, you will get thin.

What you may not know is that in addition to the predictable roller coaster pattern, diets are actually harmful to your health and well-being. Yes, you heard us correctly: diets are *hazardous* to your health. The problem with diets is not just that they don't work—as if that weren't enough—but that they actually have detrimental side effects.

In an article in the *New England Journal of Medicine* entitled "Losing Weight—An Ill-Fated New Year's Resolution" (1998, 338:52–54), Jerome P. Kassirer, MD, and Marcia Angell, MD, assert: "There is a dark side to this national preoccupation. Since many people cannot lose much weight no matter how hard they try, and promptly regain whatever they do lose, the vast amounts of money spent on diet clubs, special foods, and over-the-counter remedies, estimated to be on the order of $30 billion to $50 billion yearly, is wasted. More important, failed attempts to lose weight often bring with them guilt and self-hatred. After all, even overweight people are likely to share common prejudices about themselves as lazy, undisciplined, and self-indulgent. To add injury to insult, the latest magical cures are neither magical nor harmless…until we have better data about the risks of being overweight and the benefits and risks of trying to lose weight, we should remember that the cure…may be worse than the condition."

Research bears this out. There is more and more evidence that diets pose an increased risk for weight gain, weight cycling and disease, eating disorders, and depression.

Diets Make People Fatter

With each diet, the body will defend itself by fighting against restriction and weight loss for its own survival. As will be discussed in later sections, our physiology has been programmed through evolution and adaptation to respond to times of famine in ways that maximize species survival. Our bodies are wired to fight against weight loss! Each time the body defends itself against a diet, it becomes more efficient at storing fat. Studies have repeatedly revealed that compared to their non-dieting counterparts, dieters are more likely to *gain* weight in the long run. In fact, David Garner, an eating disorder specialist, has explained that the best way to gain weight is to go on a diet to lose weight!

Weight Cycling and Disease

The common response to a failed diet is to begin yet another weight loss plan, moving the dieter into a weight cycling paradigm. Along with the emotional toll of losing and regaining weight are the physical risks associated with yo-yo dieting. Glen Gaesser, author of *Big Fat Lies:*

The Truth about Your Weight and Your Health, points out that the vast majority of dieters, whose weight fluctuates considerably throughout their adult lives, have a greater risk of health problems. For example, the risk for cardiovascular disease and type 2 diabetes increased for yo-yo dieters as compared to their non-dieting counterparts, who maintained higher but steady weights.

Eating Disorders

Dieting behavior is an important predictor in the development of an eating disorder. People who diet are eight times more likely to develop bulimia or anorexia nervosa, the latter of which has the highest fatality rate of any psychiatric illness. The prevalence of eating disorders has continued to increase. In the United States, as many as ten million females and one million males struggle with an eating disorder.

Depression

Dieting poses serious physical consequences, but it also contributes to psychological problems. The effects of caloric restriction include depression, fatigue, weakness, irritability, social withdrawal, and reduced sex drive. Debra Waterhouse, dietician and author of *Why Women Need Chocolate,* notes the physiological effects of dieting that can lead to emotional consequences. She explains that dieting causes brain turbulence by decreasing brain chemicals and brain sugar supplies, which results in increased food cravings and depressed mood. Dieting decreases serotonin levels, which are needed in order to maintain a calm and stable mood. Studies of adults have found that the more diets women had been on, the more severe their depressive symptoms were. Dieters score higher on measurements of stress and depression compared to non-dieters. Dieting affects a person's emotional life negatively and inhibits a positive connection between mind, body, and spirit.

Shame

Dieters are attempting to lose weight and improve their lives. Yet diets actually worsen the very problem they are meant to solve. The long-term effects of dieting for the great majority of people are decreased health and increased weight. But perhaps the most insidious part of the whole cycle is the underlying and persistent feeling that something must be wrong with you, that you are to blame.

Have you felt it, that deep, pervasive experience of self-loathing that seeps into the core of your being? It's present when you flip through a fashion magazine, get dressed for an evening out, or get on the scale. It's there when you walk into a crowded room, shop for clothes, or see family after you have gained weight. And it's there every time you inevitably break a diet. It's the feeling of shame.

We live in a society that places emphasis on outward appearance and equates beauty, health, and success with attractiveness. Today, attractiveness is defined as being thin—very thin. This thin ideal is unattainable by the great majority of the population, but the enormous diet industry insists that with enough willpower and products *du jour,* you could be one of the lucky few chosen from the undesirable masses. In a culture that refuses to acknowledge that healthy, beautiful bodies come in all shapes and sizes and that insists that dieting can make you permanently thin, a lot of people are walking around feeling that something is terribly wrong with their bodies and themselves.

Dieters of all sizes feel their body is unacceptable because it fails to meet the societal view of perfection, which ultimately doesn't exist. The airbrushed, computer-generated, touched-up models to whom we are taught to compare ourselves ensure that we can never truly measure up.

The truth is we live in a shame-based culture that says that if your body differs from the coveted thin physique, something is intrinsically wrong with you and in need of fixing. Your worth as a person has become inaccurately defined and simplified as thin equals a good, moral person and fat equals a bad, shameful person. The words people use in everyday speech show how much we have taken this equation to heart. Have you ever said these statements to yourself?

- I was bad today (referring to what you ate).
- I'm embarrassed to go out because I feel too fat.
- I've let myself go.
- I'm ashamed to eat in public.
- I'm too ashamed to be seen in public.

These are shaming statements that go to the core of how we experience ourselves. The result is that you feel nothing about you is okay.

- You feel you are what you weigh and let the scale determine your worth.
- You envy thin people and equate their appearance with every manner of success, while your body implies failure.
- You feel "less than" because of your body size.
- You feel that if only you could lose weight and get thin, all of these negative feelings would disappear.

If you see yourself in these statements, it means that the shame-based cultural messages have been incorporated into your very identity. Rather than seeing the culture at fault for its insistence that only one type of body is acceptable, you have adopted the faulty belief that "I am flawed and defective because I am not thin enough and haven't been able to get and stay thin through dieting."

Accepting the Shame–Based Culture into Your Psyche

The consequences of these beliefs are enormously damaging to one's physical, emotional, and spiritual well-being. The process is a dangerous downward spiral. Again, because this process is experienced by virtually everyone embarking upon a diet, it must be seen as the natural progression of a set of circumstances, rather than the problem of a particular individual. The first step is absorbing a culturally induced body hatred into your psyche. It is only because you live in a culture that induces feelings of shame for not being thin enough that you embark upon a diet in the first place. The act of dieting mirrors the notion that you are either a good person because you are dieting or a bad person because you have broken your diet.

Next, once you have taken in these shame-based cultural messages, it is understandable that you turn to diets to lose weight so you can lose the shame. The problem is that the culturally supported idea of dieting to lose weight doesn't work—at least for the long term. Remember, 95 to 98 percent of all dieters will gain back their weight. When the pounds return, you are left feeling like a diet failure. After all, the prevailing "wisdom" is that if you had had enough determination, you would have kept the weight off.

Despite the fact that this is based on myth rather than fact, you are left feeling that regaining the weight is a testament to your lack of willpower and weak self. You feel *ashamed* that you have not changed your body in the way you feel you must in order to be happy and successful. You feel *disgusted* with yourself as you continue to binge on "forbidden" foods before you begin yet another diet. The anger that surfaces is directed at yourself as a failure, rather than at the culture that at its roots is shame-based when it comes to body size. When you begin looking at your body as a negative object that must be manipulated into something more acceptable and adopt dieting as the method to achieve this goal, you have taken in the culturally induced shame as your own. When you berate yourself because the diet fails, believing you are at fault and experiencing a profound sense of shame, you have taken in the culturally induced shame and made it your personal shame.

As you repeat this process, you find yourself in the diet/binge cycle, feeling ashamed and believing there is no one to blame but yourself. You believe that your shame originates from a personal source, a flawed body and character, rather than originating from a culture that creates the shame and offers the solution of dieting, which fails almost every time. By becoming aware of the dynamics of shame, and how shame moves from cultural messages into the very depths of your core identity and being, you can gain power over it.

When you name these cultural messages as the form of oppression they are, you can begin the process of healing. You can begin to challenge the notion that only one body type is acceptable and that dieting is a healthy method to achieve that body. You can begin to celebrate and honor the diversity of body types and learn a new method of eating that nourishes you physically, emotionally, and spiritually.

You are entering the world of the diet survivor, and the pages of this book will reaffirm the fact that it is not your fault that diets have failed. As a diet survivor, you will come to experience joy, not shame, in your relationship with food, your body, and yourself. You are embarking on a healing process that is life-affirming rather than life-destroying. We honor you and are glad that you are here.

Identifying the Culprit

*"Thank you for calling the Weight Loss Hotline.
If you'd like to lose a half pound right now,
press the number one 18,000 times."*
—Randy Glasbergen

D ieting has become one of the great American pastimes. You read about the latest diet craze, enter weight loss contests, talk about your dieting struggles, celebrate the shedding of pounds, and commiserate about their eventual return. As you get in the grocery checkout line, tabloids bombard you with headlines about an actress who dieted her way to slenderness and another whose weight "ballooned." As you unload your shopping cart, magazine covers promise that you can lose weight and keep it off, that you can have firm abs and thin thighs, and that you can accomplish all of this before the spring fashion season rolls in. The nightly news broadcasts updates and bulletins about the promise of a new diet regimen, the dangers of a fallen diet regimen, and the constant quest to find the perfect diet regimen. The world of dieting is a given in your life, as normal as the rising of the sun in the east and its setting in the west. It is almost impossible to imagine living any other way than contemplating starting a diet, being on a diet, or breaking a diet. Underneath the weight loss frenzy is the conviction that with any diet, it is ultimately a question of willpower, strength, and determination that will render you successful in your quest to be thin.

Pursuing the American Dream

It is no coincidence that these are the traits that are valued so greatly in the dieting culture, as they mirror the highly valued qualities embedded in society at large. They are the traits that are told in the tales of those who achieved the American Dream. The notion of pulling yourself up by your bootstraps and the idea that with enough hard work, perseverance, determination, and commitment you can achieve success, are the stories upon which this nation was founded. Those who achieved such positions, the political and economic elite, have had great influence on the shaping of beauty ideals at various points in time as a reflection of who has achieved "success" and who has not.

In the late 1800s, a full, plump body was a sign of health and prosperity. Having a round, fat body signaled that a person had achieved a high level of financial success and could afford to eat well. As the agricultural economy of that time moved into the industrial revolution, immigrants came to this country to find work. Many of these immigrants were genetically shorter and rounder than the early American settlers who were of Northern European descent. Cities became heavily populated as people sought out jobs. With the advent of railroads and refrigeration, large companies that were now processing food could distribute these goods to a greater number of people. Food became abundant and available to all but the poorest. When great numbers of people of modest means were able to become plump, and when so many immigrants naturally fell into this body type, members of the financially well-to-do wanted to distinguish themselves and their financial success from the rest of society. The signs of prestige shifted. People who were rounder were seen as common and inferior, and being thin became a sign of wealth. After all, the concept of an ideal is always in relation to what most people cannot attain. Once a majority of people develop that characteristic, it is no longer idealized.

The Western ideal of thinness has now been exported across the world. Today, being thin is a symbol of success. Take a moment and think about what that means for you. When you see a thin person or think about yourself at a lower weight, what are the attributes you associate with that body type? What about when you see a fat person or see yourself at a higher weight? Do the qualities you imagine differ, depending on the body type? In this culture, being thin or fat is fraught with notions that go far beyond differing body types.

Thin and fat have become code words full of meaning, and the national pursuit of slenderness has reached a point where the character of a person is deduced from the size of his or her body. If the origin of the American

Dream is about attaining a certain level of economic success *regardless* of one's initial circumstances, attaining the American Dream in the physical realm means getting and staying thin *regardless* of one's initial circumstances, that is, body type. Just as the American Dream promises that in this land of equality and opportunity, with enough self-reliance, hard work, and determination everyone can achieve economic success, so too have we been taught that this holds true in the realm of dieting.

Over the years it became apparent that while the American Dream was held out as the reward for those who exemplified those highly regarded qualities, not everyone who was determined, worked hard, and persevered attained economic success. The fact that inequities existed within the system, which impacted on one's ability to succeed, ultimately led to the involvement of the judicial and legislative branches of our government in an effort to address an uneven playing field.

It's Not Mind Over Matter

We are here to tell you that that as a dieter, you are on an uneven playing field. Despite the fact that you are *determined* to lose weight, that you have *worked hard* to stay thinner, and that you have shown *perseverance* in your dieting attempts, not all bodies are created equally in size and shape. In this current climate of "thin is in," everyone is clamoring to reach this ideal, this American Dream represented by this body size. But we are all starting at different points on a continuum. Some people are naturally thin while others are naturally larger. Some people are short while others are tall. Body size is less malleable than the current beliefs about dieting would have you believe. In fact, it is estimated that between 50 to 80 percent of our weight is due to genetics, and our genes largely determine our metabolism, which in turn is a major factor in determining our weight. The prevailing notion that you can lose weight and keep it off if you just try hard enough, stay committed, and remain determined is based more on fiction than fact. But do we tell ourselves that? Do you tell yourself that?

The fact that you have been on at least one diet and regained the weight places you deeper into the physiological forces that, along with genetics, so greatly influence the body. Through evolution, the body has developed a predisposition to hold on to fat after each period of food shortage. The body does not distinguish between food scarcities brought on by a famine and a self-imposed weight loss diet to meet the current ideal of thinness. In trying to reach the American Dream of thinness through dieting, those restrictive measures actually move you closer to the American Nightmare of the diet/binge cycle.

The idea that dieting is the great equalizer of body types and that it is possible for anyone committed to dieting to permanently lose weight has hurt countless numbers of people. Every person has a set point or weight range that the body seeks to maintain. When you take in less food, your body compensates by lowering your metabolism to conserve energy. When your body takes in more food, your metabolism speeds up. In this way, your body is able to maintain its set point range, the weight that is natural and healthy for you.

When you go on a diet, regardless of what plan, your body prepares for a famine. When you do eventually take in more food—and you will—your body learns to store fat more efficiently in preparation for the next famine/diet. This is why dieting so often leads to higher than pre-diet weights. Far from being the great equalizer, dieting wreaks havoc on your body and encourages physiological responses that move you farther away from your intended goal.

The idea that every body can attain a certain level of thinness is preposterous. Can we all be the same height? Can we all be the same race? Can we all have the same eye color? Our bodies naturally come in different shapes and sizes, and our weight falls within a range that suits our makeup. Attempting to alter your body through dieting often results in the exact opposite of your intended goal:

weight gain. While your body is trying to protect you by fighting your diet restrictions every step of the way, you feel like you have failed by not trying hard enough. Stop. Your body is not your enemy. When did you first learn it was you against your stomach, hips, and thighs? You don't have to continue engaging in this civil war. Let's call a truce. You deserve to live in peace.

The Powers That Be

The belief that dieting is the great equalizer keeps you hooked into the prevailing notion that if only you could muster more determination, you would succeed by getting thinner. When this doesn't happen, you blame yourself, perhaps become depressed, experience a lower sense of self-esteem, and feel shame. This process ensures the continuation of the belief that permanent weight loss is possible for all who show the required attributes. By blaming yourself, rather than challenging the culture that peddles and perpetuates the myth that diet determination leads to lasting weight loss, you guarantee the cycle will continue.

But why would anyone want that cycle to continue? Who benefits from having you believe that it is your lack of willpower that accounts for your diet failure? That it is your lack of resolve and hard work that accounts for the return of the pounds?

How many advertisements for weight loss pills, supplements, teas, and creams do you read about in a day, a week, or a month? How many television commercials implore you to do something *now* about your weight? Weight loss programs repeatedly present a before and after picture of a person who was unhappy, lethargic, and fat, but after embarking on the program or diet plan being advertised, the person is now happy, energetic, and thin. In such a short time! Her life has turned around! What are you waiting for? This could be you! Order now! Of course, each commercial or advertisement now runs a very tiny disclaimer on the bottom of the ad. It reads, "Results are not typical." We want to put it out there so everyone can read this without a magnifying glass. RESULTS ARE NOT TYPICAL! But the disclaimer is either so small, or run sounbeliev-ablyquickly, that viewers—the potential consumers—are left with the feeling that they too can achieve "success" with this product. They too can be thin, with the promise of happiness ever after.

In 1989, the Federal Trade Commission, in charge of regulating advertising and marketing, began investigating commercial weight loss claims. From 1992 to 1993, it charged seventeen companies, including the five biggest in the United States—Weight Watchers, Jenny Craig, Nutri/Systems, Physicians Weight Loss Center, and Diet Center—with making false and deceptive claims about both the safety and efficacy of their programs. They discovered that less than 1 percent of people are able to maintain weight loss for five years, despite the companies' insistence that their programs were effective. Moreover, leading obesity researchers often have an economic stake in promoting commercial weight loss programs, as they serve as consultants or researchers for or present at conferences sponsored by the weight loss companies. There are strong economic benefits for those in the diet and advertising industries to keep you feeling insecure about your body and believing that their product will be the answer to your prayers.

You continue to spend more money as the diet program or product repeatedly fails. But, and this is crucial, if these companies can convince you that *you* have failed in your use of the product, rather than the product failing you, they can become and remain successful.

The diet and advertising industries are taking advantage of the values embedded in the American Dream. The idea that we can accomplish anything with the right attitude and values keeps us trying over and over again. This reasoning fails to address the impact of genetics, physiology, and evolution in matters of body size and weight. Of course, there are choices that each individual can make regarding food, activity, and lifestyle, but even if everybody ate the exact same foods and engaged in the same amount of daily activity, there would still be a wide variation of body sizes.

Ending the Exploitation

We live in a nation that embraces the idea of a melting pot. We are a country that purports to celebrate the different races and ethnicities that together have made this country a blending of peoples, ideas, and cultures. It is time to embrace the idea of a melting pot within the area of size diversity: the celebration of different body sizes. Your body deserves to be treated with respect and with love. No one has the right to tell you that your body is somehow "less than" because of the temporary cultural idealization of one body type at the expense of all others. No one has the right to take advantage of you by insisting that you are flawed and in need of fixing. No one has the right to claim that if you pay the price, both financial and personal, you will be transformed into some preconceived notion of acceptability. No one has the right to blame you when the desired changes fail to happen, because the failure is in the product itself.

The weight loss advertisers know that their products won't work, and that's why they have to include the disclaimer. Allow yourself a moment to take that in. You are not to blame, and you have been taken advantage of. You have survived in a land abundant with diet and weight loss myths, fertile with products and gimmicks. Allow yourself to raise your voice and say no to the manipulation, no to the false promises. You have the right to life, liberty, and the pursuit of happiness at any body size. As a diet survivor, you have the opportunity to determine your own truth and decide how you want to live your life. Giving up dieting is hard. It's hard to let go of the fantasy that the perfect diet is out there and that if you follow it perfectly you can have the perfect body and the perfect life. What we present in the pages that follow is the space to experience living fully and freely in your body without the preoccupation of dieting and weight. We invite you to embark on a journey to yourself, where there are no products you must buy and no hidden disclaimers. We know it can be scary to leave the familiar, even when the familiar is problematic, but by ending the dieting cycle, you can begin to reclaim your life.

3

Reclaiming Your Life

*"And the day came when the risk it took
to remain tight in the bud was more painful
than the risk it took to blossom."*

—Anaïs Nin

Information and knowledge translate into power. For years, the cultural messages have insisted that it is your fault that your dieting attempts have failed. But you are not to blame. With an understanding of why diets fail, you can become empowered and reclaim your life.

Taking back your life means establishing a normal relationship with food. It means reaching a place of acceptance with yourself and your body. And it means taking very good care of your needs. The path to taking back your life is actually quite simple. Imagine this: eating when you are hungry, eating what you are hungry for, and stopping when you are full. This is your birthright. You were born knowing how to eat in this natural way. After so many years of struggling, it may seem unbelievable that this could be the answer. Think for a moment:

- Do you know when you are hungry?
- Do you eat when you are hungry?
- Do you eat what you are hungry for?
- Do you stop when you are full?

This method of feeding yourself, known as *attuned eating* (also referred to as intuitive eating), is based on the groundbreaking work developed in the 1980s by Jane Hirschmann and Carol Munter, authors of *Overcoming Overeating* and *When Women Stop Hating Their Bodies.* Attuned eating is powerful, and its rewards are immense. Attuned eating allows you to end overeating, to feel calm around food, and to end the preoccupation with eating that drains your mental energy.

Although we've said the solution is simple, implementing these concepts can be quite challenging at times. After all, you must contend with a culture that tells you thinness is essential. You may also contend with psychological factors that compel you to eat for emotional reasons. In addition, you must undo years of learning to ignore your natural hunger. The process looks different for each person who embarks on this journey because each of us is unique. However, everyone will experience the immense relief that comes with learning to be in tune with your own body and letting go of deprivation, from making peace with food and yourself.

Attuned eating does more than solve your problems with food; it allows you to take back your life. When you end diets and relearn how to eat in a normal way, you are in a position to make important changes in your life. As the food no longer beckons, you will learn how to deal with your feelings without reaching for food if you are an emotional eater. As you learn to eat according to your body's physiological cues, you will learn to feel more comfortable in your body and more respectful of yourself. As you learn the physical and psychological satisfaction that comes from recognizing and meeting your needs with food, you will become empowered to meet your needs in other areas of your life.

Relief and Grief

It is time to start weighing the evidence instead of weighing yourself. There is a mountain of research that identifies the failure resting within the dieting process itself, not within you. The diet is a faulty product based on faulty assumptions and driven by economic incentives. You have been falsely accused of lacking willpower and acting weak. On the contrary, you are strong; you are a diet survivor.

Allow yourself to feel this relief. It is like a warm, freshly laundered blanket on a cold night. Let yourself be wrapped in the comfort. Let your body luxuriate in the softness, resting in the knowledge that you are not at fault. But as you rest in this place, something happens. The warm blanket soon loses its heat; its comfort is less absolute. The relief that the diet itself is to blame quickly turns to sadness, to grief. You have just experienced a significant loss in your life: the belief that through dieting you could permanently change your body. *With that loss is the letting go of the fantasy that if only you could get thin, you will be happier, more successful, more loved.* You have invested time, money, and your very soul in this quest. The dieting process itself has been integral in organizing your life. The day is dictated by the food you will or will not eat. Your success or failure in following this plan determines your overall day, whether it is ultimately a "good" day or a "bad" day.

The dreariness and chilliness of a late fall evening don't matter when you've followed your diet, when your jeans fit, when you're feeling *thin.* But then again, the pink-orange melting of an autumn sky at dusk, the rustle of the maple leaves, and the smell of the crisp fall air hold little pleasure if you are yelling at yourself for eating a box of cookies, for breaking your diet, for ruining your life.

As a dieter, it is as if you have put on a pair of glasses that filter the world into all-or-nothing thinking based upon calories, body, and weight. When you are wearing these glasses, your view is constricted, and what you can or cannot take in is based on where you are with your diet. Taking off the glasses is both scary and freeing. It is scary because if you have seen the world and your place in it as being determined by losing weight, you must now look at the broader scope of who you are and what you truly want in your life, regardless of your body size. At the same time, it is freeing because if you no longer define yourself in terms of good or bad based on dieting, weight, and body size, and no longer let this all-or-nothing thinking determine what you can and cannot do in your life, you have the expansiveness of the world before you.

Stages of Loss

There are five stages in the process of loss and grief. As you contemplate the meaning of ending diets and becoming a diet survivor, spend some time thinking about where you are in this process.

Denial

You may find yourself questioning whether you must truly give up on the idea that diets can make you permanently thin. After all, research shows that diets fail in the long term about 95 to 98 percent of the time. That still leaves a tiny percentage of people who have lost weight without regaining it back. Perhaps you imagine that you could be one of those people. Why not? Maybe if you found a new diet and were absolutely determined to stick to the plan. For life. But haven't you tried this before? Haven't you had this conversation with yourself as you tried yet another diet? And did it work in the long run? Dieting is seductive. The fantasy is always dangling in front of you. It is understandable that you may find yourself in denial about the inherent failure of diets. You may find yourself engaged in another cycle of dieting before you are convinced that this is true for you.

Anger

You may lament, "Why me?" You may turn your anger against yourself by berating your body. Anger may also be directed at others. It may seem unfair that some people are naturally thin no matter what they do, while you have tried so hard to achieve that body size. Perhaps you feel anger when you see a colleague or friend losing weight and you wish it were you instead. But how many times *was* that you? How many times have you dieted and lost weight and had others envying you? This is part of the cycle; the weight is lost and you are congratulated. The pounds return and there is silence.

As you come to understand the physiology of your body, you may also become angry when others continue to judge you based on your size. They may wonder why you don't just do something about the weight because they fail to understand or accept the role of genetics, physiology, and evolutionary factors that contribute to body size and diet failure.

Bargaining

The ideas presented thus far make sense to you, but you find yourself thinking that you will try dieting one more time. You may reason that after you lose weight this time, *then* you'll consider living a life free from dieting, where you will eat in a more attuned fashion and where your worth will no longer be measured on the bathroom scale. But first you want to lose five pounds, twenty pounds, fifty pounds, one hundred pounds. "Let me just lose weight first," you tell yourself, "and then I'll quit dieting."

Depression

You are being asked to consider living your life without the goal of weight loss and its associated rewards when, up until now, your life has been focused and organized around this premise. The sadness in shifting your beliefs about the merits of dieting and the requisite of thinness is a difficult challenge. It is as if you are being asked to give up on yourself. In fact, the opposite is true. We are asking you to consider living an authentic life where your true self, that part of you that has been waiting for permission to start living, can begin breathing today.

Acceptance

You have come to a point where you accept the inherent failure of diets and no longer choose to diet in an effort to get thinner. At this stage, you understand that dieting wreaks havoc on your ability to find your natural weight range. You see the cost of dieting in both physical and emotional terms, and you are no longer willing to pay the price. You are committed to taking care of yourself in the best way you can and to allowing your weight to settle in its natural range as a function of eating in an attuned manner and engaging in an activity level that suits both your body and your life. As a diet survivor, you practice acceptance of yourself and others in their wholeness and live a life of freedom and authenticity.

These stages of loss are not always distinct, and you may find yourself experiencing two stages simultaneously or moving back and forth between the various stages.

Reclaiming Your Life

You are at a crossroads with decisions to be made about how you will live your life. To continue dieting is to take a linear path where you diet, lose weight, and regain pounds. When you embark on the road as a diet survivor, your path is more like a deepening spiral. Your relationship with food is based on the accumulation of attuned eating experiences in which you listen to internal cues to guide you.

There are compelling reasons to let go of dieting. Imagine living a life where you feel calm around food. Imagine trusting yourself as you listen to internal cues telling you when you are hungry, what you are hungry for, and when you have had enough. Imagine enjoying all foods, without labeling any as "good" or "bad." Imagine not going on a binge. Imagine your days without judging them as good or bad based on diet, food, or weight. Imagine feeling comfortable in your body and wearing clothes that you love. Imagine moving your body in ways that feel good, improving your health in the process. Imagine coping with life's inevitable ups and downs without using food to manage feelings. Imagine living in the world without feeling deprived. Imagine feeding yourself in such a loving fashion that this self-care can't help but spread into other areas of your life.

Identifying yourself as a diet survivor and refusing to live a constricted life takes courage. Challenging the societal dictates that insist upon dieting to meet the unrealistic cultural ideal is difficult. However, you can begin to change the tide for yourself, and swim in a sea of freedom. And you will not be alone.

The Diet Survivor's Handbook: 60 Lessons in Eating, Acceptance and Self-Care offers immediate and accessible support for you as you acknowledge that you haven't failed diets: diets have failed you. We recommend reading this book once through, working on the lessons consecutively, and then revisiting specific concepts as needed. Within each of the three sections you will find lessons, activities, and quotes to provide you with the principles, reassurance, and inspiration you need to guide you on your journey.

You are a diet survivor. You have chosen a new path, one that is life-affirming. As you embark on your journey, may you find support, compassion, and wisdom within the pages of this book, and within the compass that is your heart.

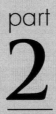

part
2

Living as a
DIET SURVIVOR

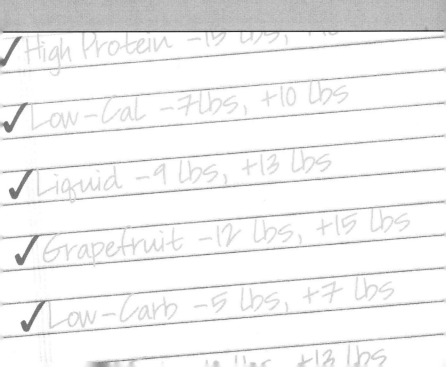

✓ High Protein -15 lbs, +18

✓ Low-Cal -7lbs, +10 lbs

✓ Liquid -9 lbs, +13 lbs

✓ Grapefruit -12 lbs, +15 lbs

✓ Low-Carb -5 lbs, +7 lbs

chapter

Lessons on Eating

"When hungry eat your rice, when tired close your eyes. Fools may laugh at me, but wise men will know what I mean."

—Lin-Chi

LESSON #1

Welcome your body's internal cues to instruct you when, what, and how much to eat.

Eating according to diet regulations leaves you in the position of being "good" when you comply and being "bad" when you rebel. Both positions are precarious and distance you from your natural hunger. As a dieter, you tried to follow the numerous rules and regulations of various programs, books, and diet gurus. When you followed these rules you felt in control, but you weren't. You were plagued by thoughts about what you should or shouldn't eat. You were trained to deny your hunger. When you could no longer tolerate the restrictions, you broke the diet rules and felt bad. This loss of control, although understandable, left you feeling worse than ever.

When you are truly in charge of your eating, you follow your own internal needs about hunger and satiation. When you remain compassionate toward yourself as you develop these new skills, you'll discover deep physical and psychological satisfaction.

As you follow this new path, the key is to shift your decisions about eating from external forces to internal cues. This process of *attuned eating* offers you a consistent and satisfying approach to feeding yourself. The work of numerous researchers, therapists, and dieticians who have studied and developed this natural approach to eating reveals that you *can* trust your body to tell you when, what, and how much to eat.

Researcher Leann Birch has demonstrated that when children are offered a wide variety of food, they can regulate their nutritional and caloric intake without parental control. Dietician Debra Waterhouse explains that cravings for chocolate serve a physiological function in premenstrual women because it helps to regulate brain chemicals necessary for physical and mental well-being. Dieticians Evelyn Tribole and Elyse Resch point out that the human body makes natural adjustments regarding nutritional needs by altering absorption of minerals and vitamins. All of this information points to the wisdom of the body to guide eating.

Attuned eating involves three steps. First, learn to recognize when you are physically hungry. This requires tuning into your stomach and noticing how it feels. Next, identify what your body craves in response to your physical hunger. In order to match your hunger with the food that will satisfy you, have a variety of foods available and withhold judgments about what you are supposed to eat. Finally, pay attention to fullness in order to know how much to eat. Tune into the body's physical cues: if you began with a signal of hunger, you will be able to identify a feeling of satisfaction when you have eaten enough. Although this process takes time, you can relearn how to listen to yourself. When you do, you will reap the rewards that come from being in charge of your eating.

ACTIVITY: Getting in Tune

1. Think of a time when you felt hungry and ate what you craved.
How did it taste?

_____

_____

_____

How did it feel in your stomach?

_____

_____

_____

2. Think of a time when you felt hungry but ate something that you weren't hungry for in order to be "good."
How did it taste?

_____

_____

_____

How did it feel in your stomach?

_____

_____

_____

3. Think of a time when you weren't hungry but ate anyway.
How did it taste?

_____

_____

_____

How did it feel in your stomach?

_____

_____

_____

Eating what you are hungry for when you're hungry gives the greatest satisfaction of taste and physical comfort. This offers a powerful incentive to eat in an attuned manner that will ultimately help you to end overeating.

"As soon as you trust yourself, you will know how to live."
—*Goethe*

LESSON #2

Honor your hunger. It's your body's natural way of telling you that it's time to eat.

A baby cries to let someone know that she's hungry. Her parent offers milk and she eats until satisfied, turning away to signal her satiation. Satisfaction is apparent by her smile and the relaxation of her body.

We're all born with the innate ability to recognize when our body needs to be fed. Yet, over time, you may have lost touch with this basic signal. Perhaps as a child you were told it wasn't time to eat, even though you were hungry. Or perhaps as a teenager, worried about being fat, you skipped meals even though your body signaled the need for food. Maybe as an adult you followed one of the numerous diet plans that moved you away from your body's natural hunger toward external rules about when to eat. Regardless of how you lost touch, you're now on the road to reconnecting with internal cues of hunger.

Your hunger is very important. If you ignore this signal, you become uncomfortable, experiencing headaches, weakness, fatigue, or crabbiness—all physical symptoms that let you know your needs are unmet. Furthermore, when you are extremely hungry, you will feel desperate and are at high risk of overeating. Begin to tell yourself: When I am physically hungry, I will respond by eating.

At first, chances are that you'll turn to food *before* feeling hungry. This is to be expected! It will take time to learn attuned eating, so remain gentle with yourself. Check in with your stomach often to see how it feels. Each time you reach for food, ask yourself, "Am I hungry?" If the answer is yes, tell yourself that this is wonderful and respond to your hunger by eating. This simple act will reinforce the stomach-hunger connection. If the answer is no, try to wait until you experience physical hunger. In the beginning, this will be difficult, but do not despair! Remind yourself that it will take time to follow internally based eating after so many years of dieting; look forward to the day when this becomes more natural for you. Allow yourself to eat, and then try again to wait for physical hunger.

By honoring your physical hunger, you'll learn that there is a way to organize your eating that's reliable and satisfying. This is the core of normalizing your relationship with food.

ACTIVITY: Identifying Your Physical Hunger

Use the "Hunger Scale" to identify your hunger. Look for signals to let you know when you're physically hungry, such as a gnawing or empty feeling. Try to respond when you feel "somewhat hungry" or "hungry." Remember, by waiting until "very hungry" or "starving," you put yourself at risk of overeating.

Hunger Scale
Starving
Very Hungry
Hungry
Somewhat Hungry
Not Hungry/Not Full
Somewhat Full
Full
Very Full
Stuffed

Tune into your stomach and notice where you are on this scale right now. If you are hungry, it's time to eat!

"If hunger makes you irritable, better eat and be pleasant."
—Sefier Hasidim

LESSON #3

Ask yourself what you are hungry for and listen to your body. Its wisdom can guide you toward a good match.

Chances are that much of what you eat has been guided by external factors. Food choices are made in compliance with or in rebellion against a particular plan. Instead, try deciding what to eat by tuning into your stomach and discovering what would feel just right to *you* in the moment of your physical hunger.

Research shows that humans are born with the ability to regulate their food intake. In fact, when tight parental control interferes with this natural ability, children are more likely to eat "restricted" food even when they're not hungry. This loss of the ability to self-regulate in children is mirrored by adults on restrictive diets.

As you normalize your eating, *you* will become the expert in knowing what type of food your body needs at a particular time. Be patient with yourself because it will take practice to relearn how to listen to your body's internal cues about what you are hungry for.

When you become physically hungry, stop for a moment and ask yourself what would feel good in your stomach. Of course, you want it to taste good to you as well, but it's important to actually imagine how it will feel in your body. It is not uncommon for people to open their refrigerators or cabinets as they muse, "What do I want to eat?" After seeing the options available, a choice is made that may or may not serve as a good match. The problem with this method is that it constricts people to picking foods that are immediately available without giving enough thought to internal signals that can help direct food selection. Try to stay in touch with your physical hunger as you narrow down exactly what would be the best match in your stomach at that moment.

ACTIVITY: Practice Making Matches

The next time you experience physical hunger, your goal is to make a good food match.

1. Ask yourself: Of all the foods in the world, what would feel just right in my stomach? Listen to your body's answer, and do your best to get the exact food you crave.

2. If you cannot immediately identify what you crave, narrow down your choices by asking:

• Do I need something hot or cold?

• Do I need something crunchy or mushy?

• Do I need something spicy or bland?

• Do I need something salty or sweet?

• Do I need protein, carbohydrates, or fat?

3. After narrowing down the type of food you want, come up with some items in that category. Which one seems best? Now, imagine it in your stomach. Is it just right? If yes, try it to see if it is indeed a good match that leads to satisfaction. If it is, you have added a positive experience to your new way of eating. If it's not, try to determine in what way you were off so that you can learn to make closer matches in the future.

"Ask not what you can do for your country. Ask what's for lunch."
—*Orson Welles*

LESSON #4

Pay attention to your fullness. When you eat from physical hunger and eat exactly what you are hungry for, you will also notice when your stomach feels satisfied.

As you learn to normalize your eating, you're likely to find that it's easier to know when to start eating than it is to figure out when to stop. Be patient and pay attention. Begin to notice how your body feels when you eat past fullness.

When it comes to deciding how full is just right, you will need to focus on your own comfort level. Think about the moment when you feel satisfaction as the point to stop eating. Some people find that the absence of hunger is their signal to stop, while other people find that they like to feel a full feeling in their stomach. You may find that the place that feels most comfortable to stop varies within a day or on different days. Check in with your stomach. Are you comfortable? Visualize how your stomach will feel twenty to thirty minutes from now. Is that okay with you? It's always up to you to decide where the line is between tuning in to your internal cue to stop eating and eating past fullness. The sooner you stop, the sooner you will become hungry again, and making those frequent connections between physical hunger and feeding yourself is the way out of overeating.

Until now, much of your eating has been unrelated to physical hunger. Remember that when there is no signal to start, there is no signal to stop. Therefore, you may have allowed yourself to become stuffed often, but you're so used to an overfull feeling that it seems natural. As you learn to eat when physically hungry, you'll find that there's a point at which you are aware that your stomach has had enough. Eating past fullness will become less tolerable over time.

An important aspect of feeling satisfied, so that you are in a strong position to stop eating when you are full, is to make sure that you eat exactly what you are hungry for. Have you ever had the experience of eating well past fullness yet not feeling satisfied? This can happen when you override the process of making a match because of a judgment that a particular food is "bad." For example, perhaps you crave some pepperoni pizza, but decide that it would be "less fattening" to eat a skinless chicken breast and salad. After your meal, you discover that you don't feel satisfied. So you eat some potato chips, then some brownies…and eventually you have that slice of pizza, but by then you're so full that it doesn't feel good in your stomach. There is a good chance that if you had given yourself permission to eat the pizza in the first place, you would have experienced the satisfaction that comes from making a good match without eating past fullness.

ACTIVITY: The Three Bears, with a Twist

Remember Goldilocks and the Three Bears? Papa's porridge was too hot, Mama's porridge was too cold, Baby's porridge was just right. Think back to a time when you felt too full, not full enough, and just right. Write down three physical sensations and three emotions associated with each experience. Reflect on your comfort level.

- Too full

- Not full enough

- Just right

> "The spirit cannot endure the body when overfed, but, if
> underfed, the body cannot endure the spirit."
> —St. Frances de Sales

LESSON #5

Become mindful of whether you are experiencing
stomach hunger or mouth hunger.

Psychotherapists Jane Hirschmann and Carol Munter developed the terms *stomach hunger* and *mouth hunger* to help overeaters distinguish between physical and psychological hunger. These concepts will help you sort out your eating as you put diets behind you and learn to trust your own reliable internal cues to tell you when to eat.

Stomach hunger refers to physiological-based eating. This term reinforces the idea that the cue to eat originates in your stomach. Each time you experience physical hunger, play it up by reminding yourself that it is wonderful that you are hungry—you get to eat!

In fact, for a diet survivor, stomach hunger indicates not only that you get to eat but that you *must* eat. This attitude counteracts some of the damage done to you by dieting. If you're like most dieters, there were times you felt very hungry but ignored these signals so that you would eat less. This behavior made you feel virtuous, in control—*and* physically uncomfortable. Although this is normal behavior for a dieter, it makes no sense!

The concept of stomach hunger also helps reduce guilt

associated with eating. Dieters spend much time feeling bad about decisions to eat, creating anxiety and negative feelings. Instead of experiencing a constant sense of doing something wrong, embrace this consistent, reasonable way to determine when to eat. Tell yourself, "I am hungry. This means I am supposed to eat!" Over time you'll find that you experience great pleasure and calmness from your ability to identify your hunger and feed yourself.

Mouth hunger refers to psychological-based eating, which means reaching for food when you're not physically hungry. Maybe you're eating for emotional reasons or because something looks good. Whatever the source, it has nothing to do with a physical need for food.

It's important to note that early on most of your eating will continue to be from mouth hunger. Remember, if you could simply read about these concepts—eating when you are hungry, eating what you are hungry for, and stopping when you are full—and then implement them immediately, you would not be a person struggling with an eating problem. Furthermore, if you try to view this as the new, correct way to eat and berate your mouth hunger, you'll only feel like you're on another diet; the Stomach Hunger diet!

Trust us, this process takes time and practice, but you will see progress. For now, focus on collecting stomach hunger experiences, one at a time. Diet survivors must let go of the diet mentality of being "good" or "bad" and instead think about a general move in the direction of stomach hunger. You'll find a strong incentive to move in this direction: you feel much better, physically *and* psychologically.

Each time you reach for food, ask yourself, "Is this stomach hunger or mouth hunger?" If the answer is stomach hunger, tell yourself that it means you need to eat, and ask yourself what you are hungry for. If the answer is mouth hunger, don't beat yourself up. Simply ask yourself if you can wait until you feel physical hunger. If you can, fine. If not, eat without a word of reproach to yourself.

Activity: Building Stomach Hunger Experiences

The idea of a savings account is a useful way to collect stomach hunger experiences. Here is a deposit slip to get you started!

ACTIVITY: The Bank of Attuned Eating

Customer # 184ME

Date of eating experience _____

Amount of pleasure I felt in the process

_____

Points of interest I discovered

_____

> *"Like an ability or a muscle, hearing your inner wisdom is strengthened by doing it."*
> —*Robbie Gass*

LESSON #6

The deprivation of dieting actually causes overeating. Making the decision to end this cycle takes courage and allows you to feel more relaxed with food.

Diet survivors initially believe that if they give themselves permission to eat whatever they want, they'll overeat their "forbidden foods." But really, it's the very act of deprivation that leads to the feeling of being out of control.

Remember that principle from science class: for every action there is an equal and opposite reaction. This holds true in the realm of dieting. The more you restrict your eating, the more you'll overeat when you break the restraints. The solution is to end the deprivation and make the forbidden foods available both literally (by bringing them into your home) and emotionally (by giving yourself permission to eat them).

A study conducted by Janet Polivy and Peter Hermann at the University of Toronto shows how deprivation causes dieters to eat more than they physiologically need. Dieters and non-dieters were divided into three groups and told that they were testing ice cream flavors. Prior to the taste test, the first group was given two milkshakes, the second group was given one milkshake, and the third group was given none. Then the researchers brought in the ice cream, instructing participants to sample as much as they wanted.

Non-dieters ate the most ice cream when they hadn't had any milkshakes, less ice cream when they had one milkshake, and even less ice cream when they had two milkshakes, in accordance with their physical hunger. Dieters had the opposite reaction. Those who had no milkshakes ate small amounts of ice cream, those who had one milkshake ate more ice cream, and those who drank two milkshakes ate the most ice cream!

The researchers explained that this occurred as a result of the diet mentality. Non-dieters eat in an attuned manner and regulate how much to eat according to internal cues for hunger and satiation. Dieters show *disinhibition*—the milkshake broke their usual restraints and caused them to eat more. Their experience, familiar to diet survivors, was, "I've already blown my diet; I might as well eat what I can now because tomorrow I'll have to restrict again."

This example illustrates the effect of deprivation. No wonder there are times when you feel that once you start eating certain foods, you cannot stop! The restrictions you have placed on yourself set you up to overeat. The way to achieve calmness is to stop telling yourself that you cannot eat certain foods and, instead, let all types of food back into your life.

At first, you will overeat to make up for the deprivation and, understandably, this feels scary. The decision to end the deprivation/overeating cycle takes courage, but ultimately you'll feel more relaxed with food. Once a particular food no longer holds that glitter for you, it's possible to eat it only when you're hungry for it. We want to emphasize that when we talk about ending deprivation, we don't mean you will eat anything you want whenever you want. Rather, you will become free to eat *what you are hungry for when you are hungry*—with full recognition that this process takes time to accomplish.

ACTIVITY: Understanding Deprivation

Imagine this scenario to better understand the effects of deprivation.

It is late Sunday evening and you have just been alerted that there is a problem with the town's water supply. In order to fix the problem, the town will be shutting off its water by midnight, and hopes to resume service within twenty-four to thirty-six hours.

- Do you notice an increase in your overall anxiety?
- What will you do, knowing that water will be unavailable for some time (run to the store for bottled water, fill pitchers, take a shower, run a quick load of laundry or dishes, etc.)?
- Do you find yourself thinking more about water than usual, and preoccupied with when it will be available?

• Do you find your thirst increasing?
This is the anxiety you experience, day in and day out, when you deprive yourself of particular foods.

"To promise not to do a thing is the surest way in the world to make a body want to do that very thing."
—*Mark Twain*

LESSON #7

When you reach for food to manage uncomfortable feelings, you are reaching for comfort. Learn to understand how you translate the language of feelings into the language of food and fat.

For all diet survivors, the deprivation caused by diets is a major cause of overeating. Yet it's also possible that there is an emotional component to your reach for food. At this early stage of the process, there is no way to distinguish how much of your overeating is due to deprivation and how much is attributable to managing uncomfortable feelings. Your initial task is to end deprivation by ending all diets and becoming an attuned eater. Once you accomplish this task, if you continue to experience overeating on a regular basis, it is likely to be caused by emotional factors.

For now, it's important for you to understand how you may translate the way you speak to yourself about uncomfortable feelings into the language of food and fat. Many diet survivors are aware that they turn to food for all kinds of feelings—anger, boredom, stress, loneliness, even happiness. However, it's not the actual feeling that causes you to turn to food. Rather, it's the discomfort you experience at the prospect of actually having the emotion that creates the anxiety that leads to overeating. Hirschmann and Munter call this a *calming* problem. Diet survivors frequently describe this reach for food as soothing, distracting, comforting, or numbing. While it probably distresses you that the side effects of this behavior are weight gain and feelings of being out of control, it is positive that you are trying to help yourself in a moment of discomfort.

Imagine that you have had an argument with your friend. You come home later in the day and eat a package of cookies even though you're not physically hungry. You probably don't say to yourself, "Gee, I'm angry at my friend and can't tolerate this feeling. I think I'll eat something to soothe myself." Instead, you just start eating. But then, you begin to yell at yourself. "What am I doing? I'm out of control. I'm such a pig. Starting tomorrow, I just have to go on a diet." You have effectively taken the anger you feel toward your friend and turned it toward yourself.

Furthermore, in this scenario you believe that going on a diet will solve your problem. This is a faulty conclusion! The real issue is that you were angry with your friend and couldn't deal with those feelings. You turned to food to manage your discomfort and then used the yelling to take you further away from what was bothering you. Dieting and weight loss will never solve that difficulty. Instead, you need to build your capacity to experience a range of feelings without turning to food. Not only will this allow you to stop focusing on diets as the solution to your problems, it will help you to stop yelling at yourself. After all, calling yourself names makes you feel anxious. When overeaters feel anxious, they turn to food. Yelling at yourself for overeating only fuels the binge!

Instead, gently tell yourself that you are experiencing distress and food is a way, for now, to take care of yourself. Remind yourself the day will come when you no longer rely on food in this way. Remember, this is a process that takes time. You've spent years engaged in dieting and overeating; it makes sense that it will take time to undo these behaviors.

Ending the criticism is key in this process. Harsh words are part of a translation to take you away from feelings and ultimately make you feel worse. By understanding this, you will be able to slow down your overeating. Speak kindly to yourself and remember to think about this as a calming problem, rather than one of food or weight.

ACTIVITY: It's All in the Translation

Play detective and decipher how the language of food and fat is a code for other feelings:

Janet has been very frustrated with her job and feels her boss is treating her unfairly. She's worried about being passed over for a promotion she knows she deserves. One day, Janet gets a phone call from her friend, who is bursting with good news about her own career. Janet congratulates her, wishing her well and promising to make a date to celebrate. Hanging up the phone, Janet begins eating brownies, even though she's not physically hungry. She begins to yell at herself about eating.

1. What feelings do you think Janet might be experiencing but not acknowledging?

_____

_____

_____

2. Imagine what Janet says when she yells at herself.

_____

_____

_____

3. If Janet decides to go on a diet because she ate too many brownies, what do you think will happen with the feelings identified in #1?

_____

_____

_____

The next time you reach for food for emotional reasons, be a detective for yourself. What feelings are being translated into the language of food and fat?

"If thought corrupts language, language can also corrupt thought."
—*George Orwell*

LESSON #8

Let go of your belief that foods should be categorized as "good" and "bad." This thinking interferes with your ability to listen to your true physiological hunger.

Until now, you've organized food into categories: good or bad, healthy or unhealthy, fattening or nonfattening. Based on these descriptions, you determine what you should or shouldn't eat. It's essential to let go of all of your judgments about food so that you can end deprivation and match what you eat with what you're hungry for.

At first, you may believe that without these judgments you will eat anything and everything. After all, there have been numerous times when you allowed yourself a "bad" food and overate. Yet these judgments interfere with your ability to listen to your body telling you what it needs at a particular moment.

Let's say you want cheese. Because you think cheese is "bad," you substitute a rice cake. How might you end up feeling? Probably unsatisfied because the rice cake is too light in your stomach. Perhaps also light-headed because your body needed the protein from the cheese.

Now imagine craving an apple. But eating an apple makes you feel like you're on a diet, and instead you decide to have a brownie. How might that make you feel physically? Perhaps the heaviness of the brownie feels uncomfortable in your stomach. Or maybe the sweetness is too intense for what you crave.

In both examples, a judgment about food as good or bad affected your decision. Our point is that, by tuning in to your natural hunger, you'll find you want a wide variety of tastes and types of food, and your selection of what to eat will balance out over time. You miss the match just as much if you eat a carrot when you want a cookie as you do if you eat a cookie when you want a carrot.

Nutrition is important; however, recommendations about what people should and shouldn't eat continue to be revised. For example, once eggs were deemed bad because they supposedly raised cholesterol. Now we know the cholesterol in eggs isn't unhealthy. Moreover, when people eliminated eggs, they lost a significant nutritional source of lecithin, which is associated with benefits to the heart, liver, and brain. Carbohydrates, once considered "good," are now avoided by a significant portion of the population. The Food Pyramid guidelines of 1992 have been replaced by a new pyramid.

Listen to your body. It knows a wide variety of foods will serve you well. Letting go of judgments helps you stay in touch with internal cues about what to eat. We have never met anyone who gave herself permission to eat and then wanted only sweets and fatty foods, which are the ones typically feared. When you learn to give your body what it craves, you'll find there's a whole range of foods that provide satisfaction and allow you to meet your nutritional needs.

ACTIVITY: Doing Away with the Notion of "Good" and "Bad" Foods

Challenge yourself to let go of the notion that food is inherently good/bad or healthy/unhealthy. Make a list of at least three foods you have considered good and three foods you have considered bad.

"Good" Foods	"Bad" Foods
1. _____	1. _____
2. _____	2. _____
3 _____	3. _____

For each food, think about why you put it in that category. See if you can think of a situation in which that food no longer fits that original assumption. For example, you might have put yogurt in the "good" category because it has calcium and is low in fat. Yet, to someone who is lactose intolerant, that food would be "bad." You might have put pizza in the "bad" category because it's high in calories and fat. But suppose you were stuck in an airport for hours due to bad weather and the only food you had with you was raw carrots and celery. Buying pizza would provide you with a variety of nutrients and would sustain you.

"Part of the secret of success in life is to eat what you like and let the food fight it out inside."
—Mark Twain

LESSON #9

Fill your home with foods you love. Knowing that there is food available when you are hungry will decrease your anxiety and provide a sense of security.

It's striking that many overeaters do not keep much food in their homes. Perhaps there is some milk, apple juice, and a few oranges. If you have a family, you may find that you buy foods they enjoy, but don't give yourself permission to eat them. Nor do you stock your favorite foods on a regular basis.

If this is true for you, take a moment to think about the anxiety that's created by not having enough to eat in your home. What is it like to walk in after a day of work and not have something appetizing available? How does it feel to imagine that you might get hungry but have very few choices to pick from? We want to emphasize that *anyone* in this situation would feel anxious. You are left with the options of going hungry, eating something you don't want, or having to go out to get something, despite the fact that you're not in the mood to leave your home. Additionally, the deprivation caused by not having enough food because you are trying to avoid eating ensures that you *will* overeat in the near future. If you go out, you had better eat a lot because there is nothing in your home if you get hungry later on.

Think about a different scenario. You notice that your stomach is beginning to feel hunger, and you think that some pasta with marinara sauce and freshly grated Parmesan cheese would make a wonderful match. You realize that you also need bread and butter. You might want something sweet later in the evening, perhaps a banana or ice cream. All of these foods are in your home. You take a piece of buttered bread to take the edge off of your hunger as you make the pasta. You feel calm, knowing that what you want is only minutes away. You sit down to your meal and stop eating when you feel satisfied. Although you are no longer hungry, you know that if you become hungry for more pasta later, you can have it. If you become hungry for something sweet, you can have it. And, if you don't experience hunger again that evening, all of these foods will still be there for you tomorrow. This is the calmness of an attuned eater. This is the security of filling your home with food.

It's natural that the idea of bringing food into your home may feel scary at first. Hopefully, it also feels exciting. If you feel ready to go grocery shopping and buy what you need, that's great. It's also okay to go slowly. Pick one or two foods that feel safe enough for you to purchase. Whatever you can manage is a fine place to start. As you discover how much better it feels to have food you like in your home, you'll be able to expand the selection to meet your unique preferences.

ACTIVITY: Filling Your Home with Food

Your task is to create a fantasy grocery list for yourself. Take some time to think about what types of food you enjoy and how you want to fill your cabinets, refrigerator, and freezer. Be specific. For example, do you like bread? If so, what kinds? Crusty baguettes? A doughy Italian loaf? Foccacia? If you want frozen waffles, are they oat bran, blueberry, or some other variety? Imagine specific dishes, such as chicken piccata or Greek salad. Explore the grocery aisles in your mind with no hurry. After you have made your fantasy list, consider how to make this list a reality.

"Food is an important part of a balanced diet."
—Fran Lebowitz

LESSON #10

Keep food with you at all times. When you experience hunger but do not feed yourself, you let yourself down.

Now that you have begun to experience the satisfaction of eating when you are physically hungry, it's important to make sure you have food with you throughout the day. Otherwise, you risk the possibility of becoming hungry, yet unable to respond to that hunger.

Let's say that you have a busy day at the office. You made a good match with your hunger when you ate in the morning. You planned to go out for lunch. However, as the day unfolds, you find yourself immersed in a project and can't take a break to get food. If you don't eat, you risk becoming physically uncomfortable. You may develop a headache, feel light-headed, or become crabby. You may even manage to suppress your hunger for the moment, only to notice that you're ravenous later in the day. Letting yourself become extremely hungry puts you at risk of overeating when you do eat and makes the possibility of matching less likely. Remember, when you are in the starving range of the hunger scale, you experience a desperate feeling in which anything will do.

There may be times when you overeat because you know there won't be any food available later. Even though you may start eating when you are hungry and make a good match, you eat well past fullness because of your anxiety about getting too hungry in the future.

The solution is to keep food with you at all times. This means packing food in a carrier that feels convenient to you. In it you can put a variety of foods that are likely to meet your needs when you become hungry. Perhaps a sandwich, chips, fruit, carrots, and cookies. Or maybe pasta salad, yogurt, pretzels, candy bars, a bagel, and some cheese. Be creative! Whatever foods you might crave can go with you. Buy an ice pack to keep things cold. Use a thermos to keep foods hot or get a small microwave for your office. Keep in mind that the purpose is to have more than just a snack. One granola bar won't help you if you need protein. A piece of fruit won't do the trick if you crave chocolate. Variety is the key.

Reflect on what it would feel like to keep food available at all times. Think of it like a security blanket—there for you if you need it. Just because you bring food with you doesn't mean that you're obligated to eat it. If you are doing errands and realize that the vegetarian burrito offered at the food court will make a better match than the turkey sandwich you brought with you, get it!

Do you feel that taking the time to prepare food for yourself is too much trouble? Does it seem self-indulgent to have food with you all the time? We urge you to try it for a while and see if it's worth it. Think about parents with a young child. Even though it may feel like a hassle, before going out they take the time to pack juice, crackers, and cereal. They know that if their child becomes hungry and they're unprepared, everyone will be miserable. Even though you're an adult, there's no reason to subject yourself to physical discomfort by waiting to eat. There's no downside to bringing food with you. You are entitled to eat when you're hungry!

ACTIVITY: Preparing a Food Bag

Do you remember the steps of those science experiments you had to do in school? We've started this one for you—now you draw the conclusion!

Materials: Bag of any size and shape filled with a variety of at least four food items.

Hypothesis: Carrying a food bag with me all day will provide me with a useful option to respond to my physical hunger.

Method: Prepare a food bag each morning. Include at least four food options covering a sampling of choices for which you might be hungry (e.g., a sandwich, candy bar, fruit, pretzels).

Results: Review your food bag experience each evening for at least one week to determine: a) how you felt having your food bag with you, b) if you ate something from your food bag, and c) if your food bag contained items that were sufficient. If not, what might you add tomorrow?

Conclusion: Determine if the hypothesis is true for you. Did carrying a food bag with you all day provide you with a useful option for responding to your physical hunger?

Discussion: Review your results and conclusions as they impact upon your life. If carrying a food bag proved beneficial, include this action as part of your everyday life. If you experienced difficulties, examine where the difficulties might lie. We have found that, while some diet survivors find carrying a food bag to be awkward at first, they soon find this practice to be invaluable. Remember, you can never go wrong with having food available but can run into trouble when food is scarce.

> *"Expect your every need to be met.*
> *Expect the answer to every problem.*
> *Expect abundance on every level."*
> —Eileen Caddy

LESSON #11

Speak to yourself with compassion. Becoming an attuned eater is a process that takes time and practice; the gentler you can be with yourself, the less anxious you will feel.

The nature of being a diet survivor means that in the past, you frequently found yourself eating amounts or types of food that you believed were "bad" for you. You condemned yourself for being weak or out of control and eventually promised yourself to be "good" again.

Each time you berate yourself for overeating, you weaken your self-esteem. You also create anxiety as you tell yourself that there is something terribly wrong with you that must be changed. But you've already tried! You've been "good" and gone on many diets—they haven't worked. What else are you supposed to do? Your anxiety increases, making it more likely you'll reach for food in an attempt to make yourself feel better. The anxiety that you experience as you yell at yourself for your transgressions actually prolongs the overeating experience. This is not a sign of weakness, but an insidious aspect of the diet/binge cycle. Just by making the decision to stop criticizing yourself when you eat, you'll find that your overeating slows down considerably.

It's important to understand that yelling at yourself will never lead to positive change. It only weakens you, making it that much harder to accomplish your goals. If yelling at yourself helped you become thin, wouldn't you already be at the weight you desire? Instead, learn to speak to yourself with compassion, which will move you in the direction of your goals.

Some diet survivors find it useful to think of the younger child within them. If this concept works for you, try to talk with the part of yourself that is in trouble in the way you would talk to a child. Or, if this image doesn't fit for you, imagine the voice of a compassionate person speaking to you. That voice may be your own, or it may be the voice of a family member, friend, or anyone else whom you experience as kind and compassionate. You may even try to imagine our voices, keeping in mind the tone of this book. Whatever feels nurturing to you is fine.

You must develop an attitude toward your relationship with food that is nurturing rather than critical. Each time you eat when you're hungry, notice the good feelings that come with this act of self-care. Each time you eat when you're *not* hungry, gently say, "I'm reaching for food and I'm not hungry. Something is making me uncomfortable right now, and this is the best way I have to take care of myself." You may even add, "It makes me feel sad that there are times I need to eat when I'm not hungry. I look forward to the day that I no longer need to do that."

Ideally, you wouldn't need to turn to food unless you were physically hungry. But everyone struggles with something, and when you reach for food for the purpose of comfort, you're making an attempt to help yourself. Wanting to do something for yourself when you are in need is positive. While using food to calm yourself doesn't solve life's problems, there are worse things people can do when experiencing emotional discomfort.

By acknowledging what is happening and your feelings about it, you create a sense of calmness. You're not weak or lazy; you're not ignoring the problems you have in your relationship with food. You are diligently working toward normalizing your eating, with full recognition that this is a process that takes time and practice. Be gentle with yourself. Learn to use a compassionate voice. As you become calmer around food and no longer fuel your anxiety by yelling at yourself, you'll notice a decrease in your overeating.

ACTIVITY: Cultivating a Voice of Compassion

List at least three harsh statements/judgments you have made to yourself about your eating. For example, "I am so disgusting for binging on those cookies. I am gross."

1. _____
2. _____
3. _____

Is there anyone else to whom you would speak in this way? Why is it okay to speak to yourself in these terms? For each statement, write down an alternative statement that conveys compassion and understanding. For example, "I don't know why I binged, and I don't feel well from eating cookies I didn't really want. Even though I don't understand why I ate them, there must be some reason. I need to be gentle and patient during these confusing times, and take care of myself in the best way I can." Or, "I am worthy of love and respect regardless of what I eat." Work on accessing that voice the next time you begin to berate yourself for eating.

1. _____
2. _____
3. _____

"Love and compassion are necessities, not luxuries. Without them, humanity cannot survive."
—Dalai Lama

LESSON #12

Learn to become patient with the process of normalizing your eating. It is important to make sure that you do not turn this approach into another diet.

Up until now, you've been learning how to become an attuned eater. You are collecting experiences in which you identify physical hunger, make a match, and stop eating when you feel satisfied. You are learning to eliminate judgments about what you are "supposed" to eat and about nurturing yourself by keeping food available. "So," you think, "this sounds pretty simple. Eat when I'm hungry; stop when I'm full. I should be able to do that." As simple as it sounds, normalizing your eating can be complicated. After all, you've spent years ignoring your natural signals for hunger and satiation; it makes sense that it will take time to relearn how to tune in to those cues. Additionally, you have to undo years of deprivation. There may also be an emotional component to the hunger you experience, and it will take time before you no longer turn to food to manage these uncomfortable feelings.

As a group, dieters often think in all-or-nothing terms. "I'm on my diet" or "I'm off my diet." "I'm good" or "I'm bad." If you are someone with this tendency, you might find yourself evaluating this approach in a similar manner, thereby turning it into another diet.

Remember the idea of accumulating stomach hunger experiences one by one and depositing them into the attuned eating bank account that you established in lesson #5? Hopefully, you can remember the moments where you experienced successes. Have you had a time where you ate what you were hungry for when you were hungry and it felt totally wonderful? Have you had a time where you gave yourself permission to eat a formerly "forbidden" food, began to eat it, and then surprised yourself by stopping because you just didn't want any more? These experiences represent the freedom that is possible in your relationship with food when you truly give up a diet mentality. Focus on the pleasure and satisfaction you feel when you collect stomach hunger experiences, and acknowledge the physical discomfort that occurs when you are unable to accurately respond to your physical cues.

ACTIVITY: Not Just Semantics

As a diet survivor, each day you'll have some experiences with food that *feel* good and some that *feel* bad. But that's very different than saying, "I was good" or "I was bad." Think about some recent eating experiences and complete the following:

Example: It felt good when I stopped eating my hamburger at the moment I felt satisfied.

1. _____
2. _____
3. _____

Example: It felt bad when I ate some french fries when I really craved a bowl of soup.

1. _____
2. _____
3. _____

"The two biggest sellers in any bookstore are the cookbooks and the diet books. The cookbooks tell you how to prepare the food, and the diet books tell you how not to eat any of it."
—Andy Rooney

LESSON #13

Create abundance for yourself. When you know that the foods you enjoy are consistently available, the need to eat because of deprivation diminishes greatly.

As you think about what foods you would like to have in your home and in your food bag, you might worry that if your "forbidden" foods were available, you would eat them nonstop. The deprivation created when you tell yourself you cannot eat certain foods actually sets you up to overeat those very foods once they become available. The anecdote to this problem, which will help you to feel calm around all foods, is the process of stocking, developed by Jane Hirschmann and Carol Munter.

Keep in mind that we want you to consider this step carefully before taking action. It's extremely effective, but you must feel committed to this guideline for the long term for it to help you. Wait until you feel ready. As you move along the path of attuned eating, always proceed at the pace that is right for you.

Imagine a box of chocolate chip cookies. You begin eating them, feel some guilt, and then decide that since you've started eating the cookies, you might as well finish them. After all, you've already broken your diet. If you finish the cookies now, they won't be around to tempt you tomorrow. Whether the item is cookies, potato chips, ice cream, or any other restricted food, this is a common scenario for dieters.

Now imagine a completely different scenario. Instead of having one box of cookies, you have eight boxes. You begin to eat the cookies in the first box. At some point you stop; it's likely you ate more than you needed, but there is no possible way to finish all of the cookies in your home.

The next day you again begin eating cookies, perhaps finishing off a second box. Again you have overeaten, but there are still six boxes remaining. You go to the store and buy two more boxes, now increasing your supply back to eight boxes. What do you think would happen the next day? Maybe you eat half of a box? And the next day? Half again? Now think about the following days. "I'm getting sick of cookies," you think. The goal here isn't to make you so sick of cookies that you never want them again. It's just that once you can have cookies when you are hungry for them, they no longer call to you in the same way when you do not physically crave them.

Please understand that we are not encouraging you to bring your forbidden foods into your home and eat them whenever you want for the rest of your life. That would be irresponsible. What we know, however, is that once you truly make all foods available and move in the direction of eating when you are physically hungry, you will have power over the foods that now have power over you.

Here's how it works. Whenever resources are scarce, human beings become anxious. This applies not only to food, but to other aspects of life as well. Think about a time when you wanted to buy the most popular gift of the holiday season. You hear that a local store is getting the item at noon. No matter what you are doing, you drop everything, make a mad dash to the store, wait in a long line, and pay more than you think this gift is worth. Now think about the same gift a year later. You know someone who would enjoy it, but it's no longer the hottest thing around. When it's convenient, you go to the store where there are plenty available at a great price. The experience is completely different. *Scarcity makes us anxious and abundance makes us calm.*

The feeling that there won't be enough of a certain food creates anxiety and causes you to eat it once it becomes available, *whether you are hungry for it or not.* After denying yourself cookies, bringing a box into your house basically ensures that once you give yourself permission to have some, you'll overeat. Given this likelihood, you may believe that the best solution is to *never* bring these foods into your home. But how realistic is that plan? Sooner or later—at work, a party, or a restaurant—these foods will be available to you. Then what? Chances are you'll feel anxious as you try to control your desire for these foods, or you will eat them and feel guilty. Neither option leaves you feeling calm and in charge of your eating.

Abundance leads to calmness around food for many reasons. Just knowing that a particular food will always be available takes away the urgency to eat it all at once. It will take some time and practice to prove to yourself that you really *will* keep these foods accessible with full permission to eat them. If you can find the courage to keep up your supply, you'll find that in a relatively short period of time, your overeating will slow down considerably. Once you demonstrate to yourself that you plan to keep all of the foods you love available for the rest of your life, you'll find, as so many other diet survivors have discovered, that these foods no longer beckon to you.

Creating abundance also means that you can no longer count on external factors to tell you when to stop eating. In our first chocolate chip cookie example, you ate them until they were gone. What if you cannot make them go away because there are always more than you can possibly consume? The answer is that you will need to make an internal decision to stop eating. At some point, you will decide, "I've had enough." Your stomach will become your guide. Remember, it's possible to make this decision because when you become hungry for chocolate chip cookies again, whether that is in one hour, one day, or one week, they're available.

Of all of the guidelines in this book, creating abundance takes the greatest leap of faith. However, the rewards of this activity are immense. When you learn to keep all types of foods around you, you'll find that you no longer spend huge amounts of time and energy thinking about food. Instead, you'll enjoy a tremendous sense of well-being.

ACTIVITY: Getting Ready to Stock

Choose a single forbidden food that you frequently overeat. Go through the following visualization.

1. How much of this item would you need to feel that you cannot possibly finish it once you begin to overeat? Don't feel ashamed by how much you might need; it is natural to feel that it will take a very large amount. (If you have trouble figuring out how you would bring a lot of a certain food into your home, such as a fast-food item, pick something that would be easier to imagine.)

2. Imagine bringing it home today. How much would you consume?

3. Is there enough left so that you couldn't possibly finish it the next day? If not, in your mind, go to the store and buy more.

4. Think about how much you would eat on the second day. Continue this until you find yourself losing interest in that food. Always remember to imagine going back to the

store and purchasing more, so that your supply never falls below a level where you cannot see the end in sight.

Does this visualization provide you with a sense of calmness? If so, even though you may feel some anxiety as well, you are ready to begin. Do you feel great anxiety? If so, wait to take this step. Continue to work on welcoming physical hunger, making matches, and noticing satisfaction. When it feels safer, then you can begin.

> *"There is a charm about the forbidden that makes it*
> *unspeakably desirable."*
> *—Mark Twain*

LESSON #14

Before creating abundance for yourself, make sure you feel ready to begin the process. Remember to move at a pace that is comfortable for you and make sure that you understand the mechanics of stocking.

Now that you've decided that it makes sense to fill your home with your favorite foods, it's important to have a good understanding of the nuts and bolts of this process to ensure success. You may find that, although this concept makes sense intellectually, you're still unsure if you can do it or if it's right for you. That's a natural feeling. As long as you understand the principles of stocking, you can begin. Over time, it will become less frightening to bring in more food.

The purpose of bringing in large amounts of your previously forbidden foods is to help you feel calm and no longer compelled to eat them just because they're there. You won't have to bring in the same volume forever; once particular foods are back in your life, stocking large amounts will no longer be necessary. At the same time, assuming these are foods that you truly enjoy, you will always want to make sure that you have some around for those times that you do crave that particular item.

When you stock, you don't need to buy large amounts

of foods that you're already comfortable eating. For example, fruit or yogurt does not usually create anxiety for diet survivors, and therefore small amounts are fine. At the same time, it's important to keep all types of food available. If you only bring cakes, cookies, and chips into your home and have no other kinds of food available, you ensure that you'll eat those foods whether or not you really want them. This will cause you to feel that you cannot be trusted with these foods, and that this approach does not work.

It's essential that you stock with the belief that no matter what happens, you'll never deprive yourself of that particular food again. It is this attitude that makes stocking so successful. If, on the other hand, you decide that you will try this method with the idea that you may restrict that food again in a few weeks or months, depending on how things go, you are ensuring that you will overeat throughout this process. The reason you will do so is that even the slightest possibility that a food may be taken away again in the future will trigger your sensitivity to deprivation and cause you to "get it while you can." This is not a sign of weakness, but a natural reaction to the possibility of deprivation. Wait to begin the process of stocking until you can commit yourself to making these foods part of your life forever.

People choose different ways to create abundance for themselves. You may feel ready to implement this approach by stocking a variety of foods. Or you may feel tentative about bringing "forbidden" foods into your home and begin by choosing one item at a time. This may feel more manageable, and as you find that the food you have stocked no longer leads to overeating, you'll feel ready to bring in an abundance of another "forbidden" food. You may continue food by food, or you may feel more secure in this process and bring in many foods at once.

Regardless of how you go about creating this abundance, it's important to keep several factors in mind. First, do your best not to judge what you are eating. Whenever you judge what you are eating as "bad," you create a feeling that you may ban that food again, increasing the risk of overeating. Second, whenever you stock a particular food, make sure that food is available to you wherever you are. If you have candy bars at home but not at work, you're more likely to eat them at home even if they're not what you crave just because you cannot get them during the day. Finally, always make sure that you have more than enough of whatever food you are stocking in order to create a true sense of security. The right amount is however much it takes to feel that there is no way you can eat it all. Then, add some more. As soon as you return to the level where you began, it's time to replenish. It may sound strange, but you can never go wrong by having too much—only by having too little.

Once you begin to accumulate some positive experiences around stocking, you will become better able to embrace this process. One diet survivor reported an experience in which she went to her pantry to eat some potato chips, and after one crunch, realized that she had no interest in eating them because she wasn't hungry. She put them away, knowing she could have them later if she was hungry for chips. Another diet survivor was surprised to find that she passed up donuts at work for the orange that she had brought with her. She understood that it would not feel good to eat a donut when her body craved fruit. At the same time, she took a donut back to her office in case she craved it later in the day. Many diet survivors describe how different the experience of Halloween has become for them. In the past, they waited until the last minute to buy candy, bought a kind they didn't like (but sometimes still ate it), or felt guilty and sick after overeating leftover candy. Now, they have candy whenever it's a good match, and Halloween no longer creates anxiety.

The purpose of creating abundance is to help you make peace with food. All foods have a place in our lives. When you are hungry for a piece of cake, how wonderful to eat the amount you need to feel satisfied with no guilt and no physical discomfort. And how nice to be able to forget about the cake when your body doesn't crave it. The biggest reason that you feel compelled to eat foods you are not hungry for is your belief that you shouldn't eat them! Creating abundance is the remedy for this problem. Keep the foods around consistently, with full permission to eat them, and you will find that they diminish in importance for you. Do this at the pace that is best for you. Always remember to stay focused on moving in the direction of physical hunger, and remain compassionate with yourself as this process evolves naturally for you.

ACTIVITY: Taking Stock

The following list will guide you as you ready yourself to begin stocking and creating abundance.

Will I begin the process by choosing one item to stock or many items to stock?

The following list includes the item(s) I will begin stocking:

_____

_____

_____

For each item listed, can you estimate the amount you think you would need to buy to create and maintain abundance? For example, if you are planning on bringing in M&Ms, and you imagine you could eat a half-pound bag of M&Ms in a day, consider buying six one-pound bags of M&Ms, making sure that your supply doesn't go below four bags. Remember, the process of stocking is to convince yourself that you will never deprive yourself again and to replace anxiety around particular foods with calmness.

"Too much of a good thing is wonderful."
—Mae West

LESSON #15

When you repeatedly find that you are unable to follow a guideline of this approach, get curious. Try to determine whether there are concrete steps to take or whether you must explore deeper.

For each phase of this process, we've discussed steps to take in order to move toward attuned eating. These basic steps—the *mechanics* of the approach—include identifying physical hunger, making matches, stopping when full, letting go of judgments that foods are good or bad, having an abundance of foods, keeping food available at all times, and being compassionate with yourself. Did you become stuck on one guideline as you're learning to normalize your eating? Your willingness to figure out obstacles will help you continue on your path to making peace with food.

Let's say that you repeatedly run out of food because you don't go to the grocery store on a regular basis. You understand that if you don't have food at home, it will be impossible to eat in accordance with your hunger. You might eat away from home when you're not hungry because there will be nothing to eat when you get home. You might eat leftovers even though they're a poor match because you don't have what you really want. Or you might eat well past fullness because what you do consume isn't satisfying.

It's extremely important that you get curious about the obstacle of not going to the grocery store. Always start by using a problem-solving approach to identify concrete solutions to your difficulty. Maybe the problem is you're very busy and there's no convenient time to get to the store. Try reminding yourself how important it is for you to have food at home. By going to the store and buying a large supply of food, you'll be able to spend less time and energy on feeding yourself. You may decide to set a schedule for yourself to go to the store on the same day and at the same time once a week. Or explore options about services that will deliver the groceries to you. Or perhaps work out an arrangement with someone else to do the shopping, providing a list of foods you require. The key is to make a plan, try it, and see if it works. If it does, you are now further along in your journey toward becoming an attuned eater. If you continue to struggle with the problem, then you must dig deeper.

Let's say that something seems to keep getting in the way of grocery shopping despite your best efforts. Reflect more on this issue. One diet survivor realized that whenever she went to the grocery store to buy more than a few items, she felt ashamed of her need for food. She imagined running into a neighbor and feeling embarrassed about the amount and type of items in her cart. Therefore, she only allowed herself to make a quick run into a store, but never truly felt that she had enough to eat in her house. And she didn't! Now that she had identified what was getting in her way, she decided that the best thing to do would be to shop at a store that was far enough from her house that she wasn't likely to see someone she knew. As she felt more comfortable buying food for herself, she resumed shopping at her local grocery store. Although she told herself that if anyone asked why she had so much food she could say she was having a party, she eventually became comfortable with the idea that it was perfectly fine to buy whatever she needed.

Maybe the problem lies deeper still. Another diet survivor had more difficulty coming to terms with the underlying issues that got in the way of grocery shopping. She did not truly believe that it was okay for her to bring food into her home. Deep down, she believed that because she was large, she should not need to eat. She related this feeling to the messages she got growing up. As the largest of four children, she was singled out as the only one who could not have dessert. Her parents offered her financial rewards to lose weight and insisted that she participate in a major diet program as a young teen. All her life she got the message that she could never be truly happy unless she lost weight. No wonder she felt that she was not entitled to eat! This diet survivor eventually understood that these deep wounds got in the way of becoming an attuned eater and therefore sought counseling to try to resolve these issues. She learned to remind herself that she was entitled to eat when she was hungry, and eventually came to believe that this really was true. At that point, she could give herself permission to eat when she was hungry, and going to the grocery store became a routine occurrence.

Life is full of struggles. We may wish it otherwise, but it is our unique histories and personalities that add to the richness of our being. Each of you will inevitably confront obstacles along the road of normalizing your eating. Don't be discouraged! When you run into an obstacle, it doesn't mean you're doing something wrong. Rather, this is *your* path. Acknowledging the obstacles you confront and working your way through them is as much a part of being a diet survivor as learning to respond to physiological cues for hunger and satiation. As long as you pay attention to the basic mechanics of this process and do your best to solve any obstacles that come along, you'll move closer to your goal of becoming an attuned eater.

ACTIVITY: Identifying Obstacles

Think about what obstacles are in your path and write them down:

_____

_____

_____

On a separate sheet of paper, spend some time writing down your feelings about the obstacles. Write freely without censoring anything or rereading as you write. Go for the heart of what you're feeling.

Next, reread what you have written and take time to reflect. Are there concrete steps you can put into action? If this solves the problem, that's great! If not, consider the possibility that this obstacle is charged with emotional meaning that deserves deeper exploration.

"Patience and perseverance have a magical effect before which difficulties and obstacles vanish."
—John Quincy Adams

LESSON #16

Sharing food with friends and family is an important part of our culture. It is the being together, rather than eating the same food at the same time, that keeps us connected.

As you work toward listening to your hunger cues, you may wonder how to handle gatherings like family meals, meeting a friend for lunch, and special celebrations. There are many strategies you can use to remain true to yourself without giving up the social aspect of sharing food together.

If you have a family, mealtimes may be an important part of your daily life. The structure of mealtime provides a wonderful opportunity for coming together to share the highlights of the day or thoughts, ideas, and feelings. It may be a time to laugh together or consider a problem confronting a family member. Unfortunately, mealtime can also be a time of tension. There may be unresolved conflicts, issues over the food itself, or difficulty in knowing how to connect with each other. However mealtimes go in your family, it is a function of the dynamics in your family, not the food you eat.

If you usually sit down to dinner at 6:30, find that you are hungry, and have prepared a dish that is just the right match, you will comfortably eat along with whoever else is at the table, assuming they are hungry! However, if it is 5:15 and you are hungry, it's important that you respond to yourself, even though you still want to eat with your family at 6:30. Eat enough of something to take the edge off your hunger so that you can avoid the problem of becoming too hungry and setting yourself up to overeat. By feeding yourself a small amount of food, you satisfy your hunger in the moment with a strong possibility that you will once again become hungry when dinner is served.

Now consider the possibility that when you followed your hunger on a particular day, you found yourself eating at 4:00. When 6:30 rolls around, you don't experience physical hunger. Can you imagine sitting at the table, but choosing not to eat? It's up to you. You can still be part of the family conversation, which is the real way in which connection takes place. Will you feel deprived? Then make sure you put aside some of the food for yourself so that you don't feel compelled to eat just because it will be gone later. However, the choice is yours. Even though you are not hungry, you may decide that you want to eat. As always, pay attention to how your stomach feels at the end of your eating experience.

Another issue that can arise at mealtimes is that sometimes people have different food preferences that affect what is a good match for them. Perhaps when you grill steaks, you can throw on some chicken for the family member who does not like red meat. Remember, it's being together at the table that connects you, not whether or not you eat the exact same food.

The principles related to family mealtimes can apply to social gatherings as well. Whenever you know that you will be eating a meal with others at a certain time, always stay in tune with your natural hunger. If you become hungry prior to the event, decide how you will respond to yourself. You can eat a small amount of something so that you do not become ravenous before the party or dinner engagement. Or you can choose to eat a bigger amount of food now and adjust the amount you eat at the social gathering. Always give yourself full permission to get your food wrapped up for later when possible so that you won't experience the deprivation of thinking that if you don't eat it right then you cannot have it later.

Food is an important part of all cultures. In addition to providing satiation, shared eating experiences give people great pleasure. Enjoy eating! As you become more comfortable with your attuned eating, you'll find that social situations provide a wonderful way to experience the joy of food on many different levels without the anxiety created when you feel guilty for breaking the restrictions of a diet.

ACTIVITY : Staying Connected

Over the next week, assume the role of an anthropologist during shared meals. Your task is to observe what is happening in a curious and nonjudgmental manner. Consider:

• Are there verbal struggles around food?
• Are there nonverbal struggles around food?
• Is there conversation between people? If so, what kind?

Don't forget to include observations about yourself. Consider:

• Am I hungry at this meal?
• Where is my primary focus?
• How do I interact with others?

Take some time to think about what truly "feeds" you and how you can incorporate your physical and emotional needs into any mealtime.

"A smiling face is half the meal."
—Latvian proverb

LESSON #17

You may find that certain foods make you feel like you are on a diet. Legalize these "healthy" foods so that you are free to eat them when they are a good match for your hunger.

Many diet survivors confront a surprising and very real issue. While on diets, there were certain foods that you were supposed to eat on a frequent basis. Common examples might include apples, oranges, carrots, celery, cottage cheese, and salads. You may find that now whenever you eat or think about eating one of these foods, you feel like you're back on a diet. As a result you avoid these foods, even if they are what your body naturally craves.

In the process of normalizing your relationship with food, the goal is to eat exactly what you're hungry for when you're hungry. If you crave a piece of fruit but resist eating it because it triggers anxiety about the deprivation of diets, then you're unable to truly meet your hunger needs. Think about the idea of legalizing "healthy" foods. Start by making sure they are available. Often, people report that because of their aversion to diet foods, the fruits or vegetables they buy become rotten and go to waste. Therefore, they stop buying them. This guarantees that when you crave these foods, you won't be able to satisfy your need. Instead, continue to buy some of these foods, even if only in smaller amounts.

Next, recognize that the reason you avoid these foods is because on past diets, you felt compelled to eat them. Remind yourself that if you decide to have a salad, it's not because you "should." Rather, it's because it is the right match for your physical hunger. *You* are in charge of what you eat. Give yourself the freedom to choose foods—any foods!—that are a good match for you.

ACTIVITY: A Virtual Trip to the Farmer's Market

Imagine that it is a brilliantly fresh autumn morning and you have time to take a leisurely stroll through a farmer's market. Notice the smell of the fall air mixing with the scent of fresh fruits and vegetables. Take time to see the array of colors: the rich green peppers, the bright red tomatoes, the deep purple eggplant. Allow yourself to sample a freshly picked Macintosh apple, a juicy strawberry, a tart blueberry.

What do you want to try? Pick a food and write a few adjectives to describe its essence. Is it luscious? Succulent? Allow yourself to bring back the joy of eating a particular food without the old judgments associated with it being "good."

_____

_____

_____

"Forbidden fruit causes many jams."
—Anonymous

LESSON #18

You are entitled to eat. Do your best not to take in the judgments of others around you.

Even as you become more comfortable with the ideas of attuned eating, you cannot help but notice the comments of others. Family members may offer you an article about the latest diet, assuming that you must want to find a plan to help you lose weight. A coworker may comment that she is "bad" for eating ice cream last night because she is too fat. Perhaps she is smaller than you and her remark makes you feel ashamed, especially if you are working on listening to your own body cues and happen to be eating a cookie at that moment. Or maybe a friend tells you that she is concerned about a mutual friend who has gained weight. These types of comments—and in our culture they are frequent—are likely to lead you back to feelings of shame and self-doubt.

It takes active work to combat these feelings and to trust yourself as you continue on this journey. It is helpful to understand these remarks as projections of the other person's views of food and weight onto you.

A woman we know who was naturally thin worked in an office setting where cakes were brought in to celebrate staff members' birthdays. She observed that whenever she accepted a piece of cake in response to her hunger, someone inevitably commented on how lucky she was that she could eat whatever she wanted without gaining weight. But when this same woman would decline the cake because her body did not crave any, someone would comment that it was no wonder she could stay so thin because she had such willpower. This woman, an attuned eater who had a naturally thin body, understood what was happening. Her coworkers placed their own feelings about eating and weight onto her. Thus, they expressed envy in their assumption that she could eat anything and everything she wanted without gaining weight, or their feeling that their own body size was tied to their lack of control over food. Whenever someone makes a comment to you about eating and weight, see if you can decipher his or her fears and anxieties, which are then being attributed to you.

Your sense of entitlement to eat may also come into question when someone you know starts a diet and loses a noticeable amount of weight. As you hear her receive compliments and see her wearing new clothes, it's natural that you may feel some distress. "If she can do it, why can't I?" Or, "How can I be allowing myself to eat macaroni and cheese when I know it contains fat?" You must remember that you have been there too. At some point, you have been on a diet and *you* were the one losing the weight and getting the attention. Yet, eventually you were unable to maintain your diet and the weight returned. While we never want to wish anyone a poor outcome, statistically the chances that the person who is now in the limelight will maintain her weight loss are minimal. While she is most likely destined to repeat the diet/binge cycle, remember that as you normalize your eating by listening to your body's internal cues, you are developing a relationship with food that will last a lifetime and will allow your body to stabilize at its natural weight.

Finally, in all fairness to your family and friends, there is a good chance that you have taught them over the years to respond to you about food and weight issues in a certain manner. You may have commented frequently that you needed to stop eating so much or even actively recruited someone to help you stick to your diet. Just as this is a new learning experience for you, it will take time for the important people in your life to understand this process. You may choose to share your goals with others or you may keep your new approach private for now. In either case, remember that the people around you have learned the same messages from our culture that you are now trying to resist. Deflect their comments as much as possible as you consistently remind yourself that you are entitled to eat.

ACTIVITY: Dress Rehearsal

Think of a situation where someone might make a comment that challenges your commitment to becoming an attuned eater. Practice a response that feels comfortable and respects your new way of eating. Here is an example:

Friend: Let me tell you about this great diet I've been on. I've lost a bunch of weight, and it's been really easy to follow. You should give it a try!

Suggested responses:

1. Thanks, but I've learned that for me diets aren't the solution, and I'd prefer not to hear the details.

2. I'm glad that you've found something that works for you. I've actually been learning a new approach to eating that's working great for me. If you're interested, I'd be glad to tell you about it.

3. I'd prefer not to discuss my weight and eating. I understand that you're concerned about my health, and I assure you that I'm addressing those issues.

Imagine a variety of scenarios. Be creative with responses, making sure to use one that feels appropriate to you. The more you practice in your imagination, the easier it will be to find the right words when you are faced with an actual situation.

> *"It is very difficult to live among people you love and hold back from offering advice."*
> —Anne Tyler

LESSON #19

Becoming an attuned eater allows you to feel stronger both physically and psychologically. The internal strength that you are building will eventually help you to manage uncomfortable feelings without turning to food.

As you collect enough attuned eating experiences, you will come to know the satisfaction that occurs when you eat according to your physical cues for hunger and satiation. You might also notice something else. Each time you respond to your hunger, you show yourself that you have needs. Each time you make a match with a particular food, you demonstrate to yourself that your needs are important and specific. Each time you stop eating when you're satisfied, you find that your needs can be met. These significant acts help you build a consistent and reliable internal structure, which is the hallmark of good caretaking. The stronger you feel on the inside, the more ready you'll be to face emotional issues.

Contrast this sense of internal calm you're developing with your internal life as a dieter and overeater. Each decision about eating was fraught with anxiety. There was constant noise in your mind as you struggled with guilt about eating too much, eating the "right" food but feeling deprived, making "bad" choices, or wondering if you should eat at all. These thoughts drained your mental energy from other important parts of your life, such as relationships, hobbies, and work. The tremendous anxiety created by worrying about food left you psychologically weakened, and therefore less able to tolerate uncomfortable feelings related to other aspects of your life. Now that you are normalizing your eating, you can move in the direction of experiencing food as a means of providing self-care, day in and day out.

Remember that as a diet survivor, you are engaged in a process that takes time. There will be moments when eating still creates anxiety; that's to be expected. The calm and satisfied feelings that surround your eating experiences will increase as you practice eating in response to physical hunger, and that places you in a stronger position to address the emotional components of overeating.

ACTIVITY: Concentric Circles

In the space below, draw a small circle. Then, draw a circle around that one and another larger one around the first two. Imagine that the innermost circle is your ability to feed yourself in an attuned manner. How does the skill of attuned eating ripple into your emotional life? Have you noticed other areas in your life where you feel calmer and/or stronger? For each circle represented, list the areas in which you notice a change in your emotional life as a result of the changes in your eating. Feel free to add circles.

> *"I am not a thing, a noun.*
> *I seem to be a verb,*
> *An evolutionary process—*
> *An integral function of the universe."*
> —R. Buckminster Fuller

LESSON #20

Once you become an attuned eater, reaching for food when you're not physically hungry signals that something is bothering you. Nudge yourself to learn more about your feelings.

Until now, we advised you to respond to your mouth hunger in a compassionate manner by saying, "I'm reaching for food but I'm not hungry. Something must be bothering me right now, and this is the best way I have to deal with it." But when you find that the majority of your eating falls into the stomach hunger category, it's time to figure out what is creating the anxiety that leads you to reach for food when you're not hungry.

When you notice that your eating has nothing to do with physical hunger, ask yourself, "Can I wait?" Knowing that your next opportunity to eat out of physical hunger is just around the corner may allow you to decide that you can. However, the nature of emotional overeating means that you frequently are compelled to go to food, even when you're not hungry. So, if the answer is no, allow yourself to eat, without reproach. Although you may feel disappointed, remember that the goal is to naturally work your way out of overeating. If you exert great control to restrain a powerful urge to eat, it will backfire and lead to more overeating.

Eventually, the day will come when you ask yourself if you can wait and the answer is yes. You may postpone the reach for food for a minute or two, or wait until your next cue of physical hunger. The fact that you could postpone eating is a positive sign of your progress. Part of what allows you to wait is the knowledge that all foods are available to you whenever you're hungry.

Because food is the earliest symbol of care and soothing, it's a common choice as a way to provide psychological comfort. For those diet survivors who use food to deal with feelings, some are clear about what types of underlying issues are related to overeating, while others are unaware of their emotional triggers. Again, we want to emphasize that not all overeaters use food to deal with feelings. Nor do overeaters have more emotional issues than the rest of the population.

To learn more about your feelings, nudge yourself in the direction of identifying your emotions. When you find yourself turning to food without a physical cue of hunger, ask yourself, "I wonder what I would think about or feel if I didn't eat right now?" See if you can notice where your mind goes and identify your feelings. Are you thinking about an incident with your child that left you feeling inadequate? Are you anticipating a family gathering and wondering how things will go? Usually, just the act of identifying what is bothering you provides some relief and calm. It also places you in a position to begin to deal directly with the problem.

If you do find that you need to eat, take some time later to see if you can remember what triggered your need. The most important guideline in this phase of your journey is to stay curious, and keep asking yourself about your internal life. Ultimately, you will need to develop your ability to manage emotions without food, and these skills and strategies will be offered in the lessons on self-care.

ACTIVITY: A Little Nudge

For the next three to five minutes, using the prompt that fits, write down whatever comes into your mind without judging or censoring. A curious mind with a compassionate stance will allow you to continue your journey to your truest self. Let your writing be free. Don't cross out or reread anything while you're writing.

• I started to turn to food when I wasn't physically hungry. I am curious to know what may be going on inside. Instead of eating right now, I'll write about how I feel at this moment. I feel…

_____

_____

_____

• I made the decision to eat when I wasn't physically hungry. I am curious about what I was feeling that led me to eat and what I may have been thinking about before I ate. This is what was on my mind before I reached for food...

_____

_____

_____

"It is wisdom to know others;
It is enlightenment to know one's self."
—Lao-tzu

LESSON #21

There's a fine line between nudging yourself in the direction of physical hunger and controlling your need for food. Find the balance that's right for you.

As diet survivors end the deprivation caused by diets, their overeating slows down. However, some overeating still persists. Instead of getting angry with yourself, get curious about what leads you to continue to eat when you're not physically hungry.

One diet survivor realized that she had legalized every food except ice cream. As she tried to understand why she was stuck, she realized she needed to have at least one food that still felt forbidden in order to protect herself if a particular feeling became too intense. The fact that other foods were no longer forbidden to her meant that even when she tried to use them to soothe herself, they just didn't work. However, ice cream continued to be a "bad" food for her, ensuring that there was something that would take her away from her true feelings in times of emotional distress.

Whatever your reasons for continuing to overeat, it's important to move at your own pace. Even as you tell yourself that you will do your best to wait for physical hunger, give yourself permission to eat when feelings are too uncomfortable to allow you to wait. During your dieting years, control was a key principle in restricting your eating. You now understand how that control gave way to overeating. A more useful way to think about your relationship with food is that you are in the process of becoming *in charge* of your eating. You are making decisions about when, what, and how much to eat in a manner that feels comfortable and respectful of your needs. Control has no place in this equation. When you stay in tune with yourself and eliminate the concepts of good and bad foods, there is absolutely nothing to control! Think about the idea of *outgrowing* the need to eat when you are not physically hungry. You're not *forcing* yourself to do something. Instead, there is no longer an appeal to eat foods that make you feel physically uncomfortable. One diet survivor described this process as organic. She found that she no longer used food to make feelings go away because it just didn't work anymore. She wasn't using control to keep herself from overeating. Rather she was reaping the benefits of months of collecting attuned eating experiences.

As you work your way out of overeating, you're likely to find that when you reach for food to distract yourself from emotional discomfort, it just doesn't work. The food doesn't appeal to you, or you just can't bring yourself to become physically uncomfortable. We refer to this moment as "the good news and the bad news." It's good news because you're no longer overeating, even in response to emotional discomfort. It's bad news because now you're left with whatever uncomfortable feelings you were trying to avoid. Of course, we don't really think this is bad news. Rather, you're now in a position to tackle your problems head-on. You can call them by name, rather than attributing them to difficulties with food and weight.

How hard should you push yourself? Only you can answer that question. Be respectful of yourself. Feeling some emotional discomfort as you try to wait for hunger is okay, but it shouldn't be so much that you are exerting great control. If you need to go to food, do so with full permission and without judgment. Find the balance in nudging yourself toward physical hunger that leaves you feeling that you are working hard enough but without sacrificing your need for emotional comfort.

ACTIVITY: Being in Charge vs. Being in Control

List behaviors/thoughts that signal that you are trying to *control* your eating, rather than staying *in charge* of your eating.

Behaviors/thoughts that signal trying to *control* your eating: Example: Because I'm not hungry, I better not eat that muffin or I will ruin everything.

_____

_____

_____

Behaviors/thoughts that signal staying _in charge_ of your eating:

Example: I am not physically hungry for the muffin, but my need to soothe myself is very strong right now. I give myself permission to eat it without reproach and look forward to the day when I can comfort myself without food.

_____

_____

_____

"Discipline yourself only to yield to love."
—Henry David Thoreau

LESSON #22

Being a diet survivor means that you'll never deprive yourself again for the purpose of weight loss. Making choices about what to eat for other reasons is evidence of self-care.

The key to attuned eating is to listen to yourself at all times. The majority of your cues for eating are based upon physiological signals. However, there are a variety of circumstances in which other factors may come into play as you decide what foods to eat.

One diet survivor rarely craved fish but thought that that it was important to her nutritional health, so she incorporated it into her eating. Another diet survivor made the decision to add soy products to her diet, while another consciously switched to whole-grain foods. Each of these diet survivors chose to make a change in her typical eating pattern because she believed it would support her well-being. Because their decisions were made without guilt or external pressure, they led to a sense of caretaking rather than rebellious overeating.

Some diet survivors base their eating on a particular philosophy, such as vegetarianism, being kosher, or choosing to eat only organic foods. As long as these choices are based on an internal belief system rather than a fear of fat, they're compatible with the concepts of attuned eating. Refraining from meat for ethical reasons is very different from not eating meat because you think it's too fattening. If you are a diet survivor who embraces a particular eating philosophy, make sure that your reasons are not connected to weight issues and that your decision truly feels like caretaking.

There are diet survivors who have health issues that may have implications for food choices. When you've made peace with food, you'll be in a much stronger position to hear dietary recommendations made to you regarding health issues and to consider how to integrate them in a manner that feels acceptable. For example, one diet survivor needed to reduce the amount of saturated fat in her diet because of high cholesterol. Rather than completely eliminating ice cream from her home, she kept some around for those moments when she felt nothing else would do and allowed herself to eat just enough to satisfy the craving. This plan kept her from overeating ice cream to make up for the deprivation she would feel if she told herself she could never have ice cream again. She also bought foods that were similar but lower in fat, such as Italian ice and frozen yogurt, which provided her with a good enough match most of the time.

Another diet survivor had diabetes and needed to carefully monitor her blood-glucose levels. With the help of a dietician who supported attuned eating, no foods were off limits to her. She learned how to test her blood-glucose levels so that she could receive immediate feedback about the effect of various foods on her body. This allowed her to learn how to make decisions about what to eat without categorizing any particular food as "bad." Additionally, she learned that because exercise has a positive effect on carbohydrate utilization, she could eat more of the foods traditionally considered "bad" for a diabetic when she was very physically active and still have an acceptable glucose-level reading. Of course, with any medical problem it is essential that you seek advice from a physician.

Eating provides both nutrition and pleasure. Becoming an attuned eater means that you end your disordered relationship with food as your enemy. Instead, you experience freedom from the preoccupation with food and a sense of calmness and satisfaction in your eating. Once you have achieved this goal, making adjustments in your food choices that feel caretaking can enhance your physical and mental well-being.

ACTIVITY: Have a Voice in Your Choice

Make a list of any foods you want to add, reduce, or omit from your attuned eating process. Then give the reason why—be sure that each decision is based on self-care as opposed to past dieting concerns. Finally, for each reduced or omitted food, list a possible replacement for any food you feel you would miss.

Example: I want to omit canned soup from my diet. The reason is I need to reduce my salt intake because of my high blood pressure. I will buy low sodium soup or experiment with making homemade soup instead.

_____
_____
_____

"I will not eat oysters. I want my food dead—not sick, not wounded—dead."
—Woody Allen

A Final Note on Eating

"Champion the right to be yourself, dare to be different and set your own pattern; live your own life and follow your own star."
—Wilfred Peterson

When you first begin this approach, you must pay constant attention to your eating as you learn to normalize your relationship with food. As you collect more and more hunger experiences, you will find—and perhaps you already have—that attuned eating becomes so integrated into your life that it feels natural. However, even normal eaters must take a moment or two to check in with their bodies and be mindful of when, what, and how much to eat.

In addition to staying mindful, normal eaters may occasionally eat when they are not hungry or eat past fullness. In *Beyond a Shadow of a Diet: The Therapist's Guide to Treating Compulsive Eating* (Brunner-Routledge, 2004), we write: "…a healthy relationship with food means eating in response to physical hunger most of the time. However, normal eating can also include experiences such as eating occasionally because something looks good, eating past fullness at a special meal, eating in response to an emotion once in awhile, or choosing foods based on nutritional content because this feels caretaking. Attuned eating means that eating for satisfaction is predominant and experiencing deprivation is virtually nonexistent. Attuned eating is a natural skill. It can be relearned by people who have lost touch with their hunger and can be reinforced and nurtured with children so that they maintain this healthy relationship with food throughout their lives."

You now have the tools to develop a normal relationship with food. It takes time and energy for diet survivors to learn these skills, but the payoff is enormous. Welcome your hunger. Enjoy eating the foods you crave. Relish the satisfaction that comes from stopping when you have had enough. Celebrate the wonderful feelings that occur when food becomes a source of satiation and pleasure, rather than anxiety. You are well on your way in your journey as a diet survivor. Congratulations!

chapter

5

Lessons on Acceptance

"I exist as I am, that is enough."
—*Walt Whitman*

LESSON #23

Respecting the intricacies of human evolution is the first step in understanding how your body responds to diets.

As you begin to work on self-acceptance, it's essential that you understand why diets fail for the majority of people.

Our ancestors were hunters and gatherers, always looking for food to ensure survival. Sometimes food was plentiful, and sometimes food was scarce. The human body had to develop mechanisms for dealing with each situation. In times of scarcity, the body adapted by lowering metabolism to conserve energy and holding on to each and every calorie consumed. Following a period of scarcity, the body became even more efficient at storing fat in preparation for the next famine. Those whose bodies were able to adapt to these scarce conditions were the ones who were able to reproduce successfully. As a species, we have inherited a predisposition to hold onto fat after each period of scarcity. To the human body, scarcity is scarcity. Your body fails to distinguish whether the lack of food it receives is due to a famine or to a self-imposed weight loss diet. The "failure" of diets is actually a "success" in terms of species survival!

During the 1940s, researcher Ancel Keys conducted a study on thirty-six conscientious objectors to find out what would happen if they were placed on a semi-starvation diet for six months. They were given food that was nutritionally adequate and that consisted of the number of calories similar to most commercial weight loss plans. The changes observed in these men were dramatic. In addition to losing approximately 25 percent of their body weight, the men experienced noticeable personality changes. They became lethargic, irritable, depressed, and apathetic. They also became obsessed with food and talked constantly about eating, hunger, and weight.

Once the men began the re-feeding portion of the study, restrictions were no longer placed on their eating. They binged for weeks, often consuming food to the point of feeling ill. Despite their overeating, they continued to report feeling ravenous. The weight previously lost returned rapidly as fat, and most of the men lost the muscle tone that they had prior to the experiment. Some of the men ended up weighing more than before the start of the study. The men's emotional stability and energy returned only after they had regained the weight.

You can now understand the predicament you've been in as a dieter. You thought you were doing something good for your body when you cut back your food intake. What you didn't realize was that your body slowed down the rate at which it burned calories, determined to make sure that what little you did consume was enough for survival and optimal functioning. You may feel angry at your body right now, but consider thanking it and admiring the intricacies of human evolution. Your body knows nothing about weight loss diets to meet a current fashion. It wants only what's best for you: survival!

ACTIVITY: How the No-Diet Resolution Is Grounded in Evolution

Challenge your old beliefs about diet and willpower with your understanding of how human evolution affects the dieting process. Respond to the following statement:

When I restrict food for weight loss, my body should respond by:

What the dieter is taught to believe

_____

_____

_____

What human evolution programmed the body to do

_____

_____

_____

"Our own physical body possesses a wisdom which we who inhabit the body lack. We give it orders which make no sense."
—Henry Miller

LESSON #24

Your genes determine much of your body shape and size. Respect your genetic inheritance.

It's important to understand the role of genetics in determining your shape and size. You understand that the shape of your face, the color of your eyes, or the dimples in your cheeks are inherited traits that you have for your entire life. However, when it comes to body size, this way of thinking falls by the wayside. There is a persistent idea that if you're unhappy with your body size, you can permanently alter your shape through diet and exercise.

Your body has inherited a natural weight range. Research has found that between 50 and 80 percent of weight is the result of genetics. When researchers looked at identical twins who were raised separately, they found that about 80 percent of the twins were in the same weight range. This means that genetic inheritance has an enormous impact on what you weigh, regardless of environmental factors.

Metabolism, which plays a significant role in weight maintenance, is also greatly influenced by your genetic makeup. Researchers estimate that between 40 to 80 percent of resting metabolic rate is inherited. Resting metabolic rate refers to the amount of energy the body burns when not engaged in physical activity. This rate accounts for approximately 70 percent of the fuel burned each day.

Your body inherits a natural weight range or set point. Your set point is where your body settles when you are eating in response to physiological hunger and engaging in some amount of physical activity. Your natural weight is not necessarily the same as your "goal" weight. You may have an idea about what you would like to weigh, but that weight is often based on cultural ideals as opposed to what is healthy, natural, and possible for your particular body. Your weight can also be affected by medical issues such as thyroid problems, polycystic ovary syndrome (PCOS), or medication in which weight gain is a side effect.

Despite attempts to alter your natural weight, your body is persistent. Like a thermostat, natural body weight has a point it will seek to maintain. When you take in less food as fuel, your body attempts to deal with this reduction by slowing down to conserve energy. Your metabolism is lowered, reducing the rate at which calories are burned. Within twenty-four to forty-eight hours of beginning a calorie-restricted diet, metabolic rate decreases 15 to 30 percent. Your body has successfully slowed itself down to defend against this self-imposed famine. Going on a diet automatically lowers your metabolism every time. On the other hand, when your body takes in more food as fuel than it needs, your metabolism speeds up and burns calories more quickly. In this way, your set point is maintained.

If you try to alter your natural weight by dieting, your body reacts to the perceived famine by feeding off fat and muscle. Muscle is the part of your body that is metabolically active. The more muscle you have, the more calories you burn in energy expenditure. The less muscle you have, the lower your metabolism, which means that fewer calories are burned. Since every diet leads to some muscle loss, as a dieter, you are placed in a position of burning fewer calories. This makes it easier for you to gain weight, resulting in an even higher fat-to-muscle ratio. Repeated dieting attempts may significantly shift your percentage of body fat over time. This is why so many diet survivors report that they weigh more now than before they ever began to diet.

Along with a lowered metabolism, your body defends itself against calorie restriction by instructing fat cells to store more fat in anticipation of a future famine. Urgent demands are sent out for you to eat by increasing your appetite. You are engaged in a battle that cannot be won from a physiological standpoint.

Because our culture holds one body type above all others, many people learn to feel bad about their size and try repeatedly to alter their bodies in various ways. The diet and advertising industries will continue to try to sell their products by promoting the idea that bodies are malleable and can be changed at will. As a diet survivor, you can reject these faulty messages. By acknowledging the power of your genes, you can begin to accept the way in which your body is so exquisitely designed.

ACTIVITY: A Picture Is Worth a Thousand Words

Embrace your genetic inheritance. Dig out old photo albums and see how your body resembles others in your family. As you look through the photographs, think about the following questions:

• Who do I most resemble in my family?

_____

• What seems to be predominant through the generations?

_____

• Does my body type reflect the majority of my family members?

_____

"And remember, no matter where you go, there you are."
—*Confucius*

LESSON #25

Cherish your body and its uniqueness. People naturally come in different shapes and sizes.

Imagine a baby in her crib, exploring her fingers and toes. Think about the joy she experiences in her body. Now look in the mirror—how do you feel about your own body at this time in your life? Chances are that the natural pleasure your body once gave you has been tarnished by negative feelings or shame about your current shape and size.

We are not born believing that one body type is inherently better than another. Rather, these ideas are shaped by the culture and reinforced in the media. Across cultures and at different times in history, different body types are valued over others. The key is to appreciate the beauty and function of your own body. Just as there are variations in hair and eye color, it shouldn't be surprising that other parts of our bodies, such as thighs, stomach, and buttocks, vary tremendously from person to person.

Changing your belief that a thin body is inherently better than a round body takes time and effort. Only 3 to 5 percent of the population can achieve the image presented by models in magazines and on television. In fact, the concept of an ideal body size is based on the reality that very few people can actually achieve it! Accepting size diversity is an important step toward making peace with your body and living more fully. By celebrating different body shapes and sizes, you can value both your uniqueness and the uniqueness of others.

ACTIVITY: A Visit to the Art Museum

Take an afternoon to stroll through an art museum. Take in the work of masters such as Rubens, Gauguin, and Botero. (If you do not live near a museum, go to your library and look through an art book.) Notice the various body types of women in the paintings.

• How do you feel when you look at their beauty?

_____

• Do any of these images reflect your body type?

_____

• Do any of these images reflect the current idealized body type?

_____

• How can you use these paintings to sustain your journey toward acceptance?

_____

"Art arises when the secret vision of the artist and the manifestation of nature agree to find new shapes."
—Kahlil Gibran

LESSON #26

Challenge the notion that thinness equals health. You cannot tell much about anyone by the size of his or her body.

Two women are walking down the street; one is thin and the other is fat. If you were told that one of these women is an aerobics instructor and one of these women struggles with high blood pressure, would you be able to determine who was who by looking at them?

When asked this question, most people said the fat person struggled with high blood pressure and the thin person was the aerobics teacher. In fact, the opposite was true.

The idea that thinness equals health is a relatively recent notion. In the 1940s, a biologist named Louis Dublin, working with Metropolitan Life Insurance Company, developed the "Ideal Weights" chart. Despite serious flaws in his research, such as collecting self-reported weights of white men in their twenties only once, the chart greatly influenced the current thinking that equates thinness with health and fatness with disease. Dublin claimed his statistical research demonstrated a relationship between increased weight and mortality rates, and he spent his life warning all Americans, including women and ethnic groups who were not part of his research, that the greatest risk to health was being overweight.

Today's health policies promote this belief despite an abundance of research to the contrary. For example, the current guidelines use Body Mass Index (BMI) to define normal weight and suggest that anything over that range is a health risk. But the veracity of this isn't borne out in the research. Height/weight charts and BMI measurements fail to take into account a person's set point or natural weight. They also don't measure the quality of a person's diet or her activity patterns, both factors that can affect overall health.

While people assume that it's more dangerous to be fat than to be thin, long-term studies show that individuals in the *lowest* weight category are at greatest risk, those in the highest weight category are also at risk, while those in the average to above average ranges are at the least risk in terms of premature mortality.

Fitness has been shown to improve health and increase longevity, regardless of body size and weight. Steven Blair, director of research at the Cooper Institute for Aerobic Research in Dallas, has challenged the idea that body size is a predictor of health. His research included 26,000 men and 8,000 women between the ages of 20 to 90 over a ten-year period. He has repeatedly demonstrated that a person's physical fitness level is far more important than weight. For example, Blair reports that obese-fit men and lean-fit men both have low death rates and that the obese-fit men had premature death rates half that of lean-unfit men.

Blair reports that health risks commonly associated with being fat are actually due to a sedentary lifestyle and a nutritionally inadequate diet. In support of his work, he demonstrates the fact that diseases commonly associated with higher weights, such as hypertension, diabetes, and blood lipid disorders, can be controlled with moderate exercise, *even when no weight loss occurs.* Moreover, his research has found that men actually increase their risk for heart disease, hypertension, and diabetes by dieting regularly.

The truth is that all we can really know about a person based on weight is whether they are thin, average, or fat. These observations are merely descriptive in nature and cannot tell you whether the person is in good health or struggles with medical issues. Let go of the idea that your health is dependent on your weight.

ACTIVITY : Take the Challenge

In our culture, we've learned to make assumptions about a person based on body size. Challenge yourself to see what associations you may be making.

When I see a thin person I assume he/she is:

_____

_____

_____

When I see a fat person I assume he/she is:

_____

_____

_____

List at least three people in your life who don't fit those assumptions.

1. _____

because _____

2. _____

because _____

3. _____

because _____

"Trust not too much to appearances."
—Virgil

LESSON #27

Weight cycling has negative consequences.
Understand the physical and emotional benefits that
come with ending diets.

Diets have a 95 to 98 percent failure rate. If you're like most people, rather than using this statistic as proof that diets don't work, you blamed yourself and tried to diet once again with even more determination. This behavior put you in a cycle of yo-yo dieting. It's important to understand the very real consequences of letting your weight fluctuate up and down as the result of repeated weight loss attempts.

Yo-yo dieters end up with increased risks for health problems, such as higher blood pressure, heart disease, and type 2 diabetes. The Framingham Heart Study included a thirty-two-year analysis of over 3,000 men and women. Those with high fluctuations (many weight changes or large weight changes) were 25 to 100 percent more likely to develop heart disease and die prematurely. These results occurred in all individuals whose weights cycled, regardless of whether they were thin or fat at the beginning of the study, and held true when other factors were controlled, including physical activity and smoking.

People with higher weights are usually encouraged to diet in order to be "healthy." Yet, the very act of dieting may be the real culprit in creating increased health risks. So far, there is *no* diet proven to have lasting results; dieting all but ensures that you will get caught in this yo-yo cycle. If many of the health issues attributed to weight are actually the result of yo-yo dieting, then the intervention you used to help yourself actually hurt you. As a diet survivor, you're taking yourself out of this unhealthy cycle and letting your body stabilize at its natural weight.

There are emotional consequences to weight cycling as well. When you begin a diet, you do so with the belief that weight loss will make you feel better. But when the pounds return, you find yourself feeling worse than ever. Surveys have shown that the more diets women have been on, the more depressed they are. This makes sense because feelings of shame intensify each time you blame yourself for a diet's failure.

As you make the decision to break this vicious cycle, you can feel reassured that research supports the notion that a non-diet approach leads to improved physical and emotional well-being. In a 2002 study, researcher Linda Bacon compared a traditional diet program with a non-diet approach. Both groups showed similar improvements in metabolic fitness, psychological factors, and eating behavior. However, the drop-out rate for participants in the diet group was 41 percent, compared to 8 percent in the non-diet group. While there was short-term weight loss and improved self-esteem for the diet group, these results were *not* maintained after one year. Conversely, members of the non-diet group showed improved self-esteem one year after treatment.

In 2005, a two year follow-up to Bacon's study appeared in the *Journal of the American Dietetic Association.* Participants in the non-diet group maintained weight and sustained initial improvements while the diet group participants regained weight with little sustained improvements. In the article, "Size Acceptance and Intuitive Eating Improve Health for Obese, Female Chronic Dieters" (Bacon et al. 2005, 105:929), the researchers conclude, "The health at every size approach enabled participants to maintain long-term behavior change; the diet approach did not. Encouraging size acceptance, reduction in diet behavior, and heightened awareness and response to body signals resulted in improved in health risk indicators…"

By identifying yourself as a diet survivor, you give yourself a huge gift. Ending the vicious yo-yo diet cycle will take you on a promising path toward improving your physical and emotional well-being.

ACTIVITY: Rebel with a Cause

Our culture encourages weight loss through dieting for physical and emotional health. As a diet survivor, you're part of a movement that is challenging that belief. Find ways to support this cause either privately or publicly. Examine the list below and pick at least one act to engage in during the next week.

- Don't participate in conversations about dieting.
- Don't buy diet products.
- Don't make negative comments about your own body.
- Do educate yourself further about the hazards of dieting and weight cycling.
- Do congratulate yourself for ending diets, and share your reasons with a friend.
- Do consider doing something that you had put off until you were thinner.

"I've been on a constant diet for the last two decades. I've lost a total of 789 pounds. By all accounts, I should be hanging from a charm bracelet."
—Erma Bombeck

LESSON #28

Much of the research related to weight and health is contradictory. Familiarize yourself with studies that indicate health is possible at every size.

It's hard to make sense of the changing recommendations surrounding diet, weight, and health. Everywhere you go, people worry that unless they weigh what the weight charts say they should weigh, they are jeopardizing their health. But how valid are these recommendations? In 1998, the National Institute of Health changed its weight guidelines—and overnight 25 million previously healthy Americans became "overweight" and considered at risk for medical problems.

Not only do weight recommendations change over time but so do the purported risks regarding health and weight. By becoming more knowledgeable about the studies—how the research is gathered, what data are highlighted, what conclusions are drawn, and whose interests are served—you'll be better able to analyze what is presented to you. The following examples will help you to become more critical the next time you hear a report that says you must become thin to be healthy.

The conclusions of the Harvard Nurses Study, which followed 115,196 nurses between the ages of thirty to fifty-five over a sixteen-year period, appeared on the front page of a major newspaper with a headline stating, "Risk found in women's weight gain." The article contained alarming news that women who are twenty to thirty pounds overweight risk early death, and therefore a weight gain of ten to fifteen pounds in adulthood should serve as a warning. Later, the lead author, who had made these claims, acknowledged that the increased risk was so small that statisticians considered it insignificant. Meanwhile, another article reported people who were twenty to thirty pounds overweight were *not* more likely to die earlier than an average-weight person. Moreover, the health risks of being moderately underweight were much more serious than previously realized. Yet, these results, which go against the prevailing belief that thin translates to good health and fat translates to disease, received little attention.

Several other facts expose the dubious nature of how research can be used. The lead author of the Harvard Nurses study was a paid consultant of a pharmaceutical company that developed diet drugs. The author used this study to testify at Food and Drug Administration hearings that there was a significant reason to treat moderately overweight people because of the risk of early death. Manipulating research to increase concern about weight had the potential to be quite profitable. This conflict of interest is not unusual in the field of obesity research. In fact, the National Task Force on the Prevention and Treatment of Obesity, funded by the federal government to set national health policy, revealed in the *Journal of the American Medical Association* that eight out of the nine board members had financial ties to between two to eight pharmaceutical companies and commercial weight-loss companies apiece. This conflict of interest has a profound effect on how data is interpreted. Promoting a bias to favor thinness, alarming people about supposed risks due to body size, and supporting products and programs designed for weight loss is making a lot of people rich. Furthermore, because of our culture's unquestioning belief that it is necessary to be thin in order to be healthy, we tend to automatically accept information that reinforces this belief and ignore information that contradicts it. As a diet survivor, you can develop a more critical eye regarding reports equating weight and health.

Our national health policy, with its emphasis on weight loss for health, is built upon a misinterpretation of statistics. You may be familiar with the frequently cited statistic that obesity kills 300,000 people per year. This popularized figure was based on a 1993 study where the researchers concluded that dietary factors and a sedentary lifestyle contributed to those deaths. What was repeated around the country in journals, magazines, and television was that 300,000 deaths a year were *caused* by obesity. The authors of this study eventually published a letter explaining that their results were being reported inaccurately. They clarified that obesity, high blood pressure, heart disease, and cancer were some of the side effects of *dietary and activity patterns,* not a direct result of body weight. Still, the statistic continues to be used in support of the view that body weight, in and of itself, is a measure of health. In fact, the statistic was increased to 400,000 in 2004. After much criticism regarding the way this figure was calculated, the Centers for Disease Control and Prevention (CDC) admitted that this widely publicized estimate was too high and that the calculation was in error. They lowered their estimate to 365,000 deaths per year. However, a 2005 study published in the *Journal of the American Medical Association* by another CDC researcher concluded that 25,814 deaths per year are related to weight. They also found that people who are considered modestly overweight actually have a lower risk of premature death than those considered to be normal weight. Yet despite these new findings, the director of the CDC stated that they were not going to factor in this new figure in public awareness campaigns or scale back on their fight against obesity.

The news about weight, diet, and health is constantly changing. Of course, we want to do our best to be healthy. We want to adopt practices that support our physical and emotional well-being. It's important to remember, however, that much of what we are told about the importance of losing weight to maintain health can be challenged. There's an abundance of research that shows that health is possible at every size. The Health at Every Size movement celebrates people of all sizes, encourages a trust in the wisdom of the body, and promotes health practices without focusing on weight. As a diet survivor, you are a part of that movement. By reading more about the research that supports health at every size, you will be in a stronger position to bring perspective to changing views about health.

ACTIVITY: Discovering the Health at Every Size Movement

There are many ways to learn more about the research that supports this paradigm. Here is a list of resources that will support you as you challenge traditional thinking about health and weight.

Suggested books:
Big Fat Lies by Glen Gaesser
The Obesity Myth by Paul Campos
Women Afraid to Eat by Frances Berg

Suggested journal:
Health at Every Size edited by Jon Robison and Wayne Miller

Suggested websites:
Body Positive
www.bodypositive.com
Council on Size and Weight Discrimination
www.cswd.org
Eating Disorders Resources
www.gurze.com

> *"Be careful about reading health books. You may die of a misprint."*
> *—Mark Twain*

LESSON #29

The models presented in the media don't reflect the real size of women. Learn how the media can create an image that doesn't really exist.

There is a growing disparity between actual body sizes and the cultural ideal. It's not surprising that 80 percent of American women are dissatisfied with their bodies when you consider that models are thinner than approximately 95 percent of the population. Today, the average model weighs 23 percent less than the average woman. Most Miss America contestants are 15 percent below the medically recommended body weight, meeting the weight criteria for a diagnosis of anorexia nervosa. Researchers have found that a mere three-minute exposure to photographs of models from popular women's magazines leads to an increase in depression, stress, shame, insecurity, and body image dissatisfaction.

Pressures for men to meet ideal standards have also increased in recent years. In surveys of college males, between 70 and 80 percent feel their current body shape fails to meet the ideal of the lean, muscular build. Men's magazines have an increasing number of articles encouraging readers to change their body shape through body sculpting and weight training.

How do you feel when you look at the models adorning the cover of magazines or the glossy advertisements featuring the ideal woman? You are taught to compare yourself to these images and to diet in an attempt to change your body to more closely approximate the pictures. But are the pictures even real? Models spend hours in hair and makeup. Photos are airbrushed and, with the press of a computer key, stomachs are flattened, breasts are increased, and waists are narrowed. This picture will then be presented as the goal toward which you should strive.

Sometimes, the features of two or more models may be used to create one photograph. The face and neck may belong to one model, the stomach and hips to a second model, and the legs to still another model. No wonder when you look at a cover model you say to yourself, "I could never look like that." The truth is, she doesn't look like that either. The model is a fantasy of perfection. It's time to stop comparing your body to an unrealistic and unhealthy ideal of how you should look. You deserve to take pleasure in your body and to feel good about yourself.

ACTIVITY: I'm Talking about Real Women

Consider the following chart:

	Average Woman	Barbie	Store Mannequin	Supermodel Niki Taylor
Height	5'4"	6'0"	6'0"	5'11"
Weight	145 lbs.	101 lbs.	Not Available	125 lbs.
Dress Size	11–14	4	6	6
Bust	36–37"	39"	34"	34"
Waist	29–31"	19"	23"	24"
Hips	40–42"	33"	34"	34"

Take time to look at the bodies of women around you: the curve of their hips, the shape of their thighs, the swell of their stomach. Notice their eyes, their walk, and their skin. Look around at the women in a communal dressing room or locker room. Notice the variations of women in their own skin: size, shape, and age. These are the faces and bodies of real women.

"Even I don't wake up looking like Cindy Crawford."
—Cindy Crawford

LESSON #30

When you create an environment of acceptance for yourself, you will feel more comfortable.

Over the years, you internalized messages that said you must be thin to be happy and healthy. Think about how your home reflects and reinforces these messages. You might use a scale to weigh yourself or a mirror to judge yourself. You might keep clothes that are too small as a haunting reminder to diet. Each time you turn to one of these indicators to measure your size you give yourself a negative message about your self-worth. While you might hope that these objects will motivate you to lose weight, the truth is that they frequently end up making you feel worse about yourself. These negative feelings create anxiety, and that puts you at greater risk of overeating.

The next several lessons will help you learn how to create an environment of self-acceptance. Learning to accept yourself is a positive act, not a means of giving up. Accepting yourself says nothing about what size you are meant to be or where you will ultimately end up as a result of this process. Accepting yourself means that you acknowledge that you're at a certain place at this point in time and that you're entitled to take good care of yourself regardless of your size. Taking good care of yourself means engaging in acts such as feeding yourself in an attuned manner, moving your body in a way that is comfortable to you, dressing in comfortable clothes, seeking regular medical care, speaking compassionately to yourself, and responding to your emotional needs. Even if you're not in a position to act on all of these ideas right now, the key is to truly believe that you deserve these things, regardless of your size.

Positive change comes from a position of strength, not weakness. Let yourself become stronger. We understand that you might not be ready to fully embrace your body. Start with small acts of acceptance. Yelling at yourself weakens you and promotes a vicious cycle of feeling bad, overeating, dieting, binging, and back to more yelling. Acceptance promotes caretaking and wellness. This puts you in a much stronger position to build your body-esteem and self-esteem. As you work toward creating a sense of acceptance on the inside, it is helpful to create an external environment that supports your move toward acceptance.

ACTIVITY: Spring Cleaning

Search your home and look for items that contain messages that promote dieting and weight loss. Then do a thorough spring cleaning!

Look for:

- Magazines that promote weight loss through dieting
- Diet books (including diet cookbooks!)
- Food scales
- Diet products
- Anything that has slogans encouraging weight loss and dieting

Consider replacing these things with:

- Magazines about hobbies or culture
- Cookbooks that represent your food preferences
- Books that support your life as a diet survivor
- Products that celebrate your decision to practice self-acceptance with inspirational sayings

> *"If you want to make apple pie from scratch,*
> *you must first create the universe."*
> —*Carl Sagan*

LESSON #31

When you speak negatively about your body, you inflict harm upon yourself. Learn to talk to yourself the way you would talk to your best friend.

Take a moment and reflect on what you have said to yourself in your mind about your body in the last hour. Next, think about what you told yourself while dressing this morning. If you were kind to yourself, that's great. However, most diet survivors frequently criticize themselves when it comes to body shape and size. Comments range from general statements like "I'm too fat" or "I look like an elephant" to berating a specific body part, such as "My stomach sticks out too much" or "My thighs are gross." Often, these comments are present so much of the time that you barely notice they exist until it is brought to your attention. While they might seem natural to you, they cause great harm.

In some of our workshops, we ask participants to write down any negative thoughts they have had about their bodies in the past few days. Then we compile the responses and read them back to the group. "I'm disgusting," "nothing fits me," "I can't have sex until I lose weight," "I'm bad," "gross," "a pig," "I look pregnant," "I look like a cow" are examples of some of the phrases used by diet survivors. As we go through the list, reading each statement out loud, the sadness in the room is palpable. Diet survivors realize that they are constantly telling themselves these painful messages. While it seems normal to say these things to themselves, they feel distressed knowing that others are berating themselves in this harsh manner. Through this awareness people are able to make positive changes in the way they talk to themselves about their bodies.

When you realize that your negative thoughts are persistent and cause you harm, you are in a position to stop them. Imagine yourself speaking to your best friend. Would you ever call her such names? If not, why is it okay to speak to yourself in that manner? Each time you notice a negative thought, gently tell yourself to stop. Remind yourself that these criticisms don't help you. Of course, they will come creeping back because they are so familiar and automatic. When you notice their return, repeat this process and over time you'll notice that they decrease. As they do, you actively promote an environment of self-acceptance.

ACTIVITY: Twenty-Four Hours of Bad Body Thoughts...And the Promise of a Brighter Day

- Over the next twenty-four hours, pay attention to the negative comments you tell yourself about your body and write them down.
- Spend time the following day reading your list. Be gentle with yourself as you take in the words you used to judge yourself.
- Take a few comments from your list and, like a computer, "delete" these messages. Then, "insert" a compassionate alternative.

Example:

Delete: My fat arms are disgusting. I hate how flabby they are.

Insert: My arms are big. They allow me to carry things, to reach out, and to hug my loved ones.

"Kind words can be short and easy to speak, but their echoes are truly endless."
—Mother Teresa

LESSON #32

Build a wardrobe of clothes that are comfortable for you at your current size.

If you ask dieters how many sizes of clothing they have in their closet, the answer is likely to be at least three. There are clothes that fit at their current size, clothes that fit at a heavier weight, and "thin" clothes that they hope to fit into again.

Some diet programs encourage you to hang onto your "thin" clothes in order to motivate you to lose weight. Yet, when you look in your closet and see jeans that no longer fit or dresses that are sizes too small, what happens? Instead of keeping you motivated, you wind up feeling upset, depressed, or anxious. In order to deal with that anxiety, you might turn to food. The behavior that was supposed to motivate you not to eat actually triggers overeating!

Instead, imagine opening your closet and seeing a wardrobe full of clothes that fit you, are stylish, and are in colors that you love. How do you feel as you go about choosing your clothes for the day? How does this feeling affect your day?

Cleaning out your closet can stir up many feelings. Some people worry that getting rid of clothes that no longer fit means giving up on themselves. But are they really doing you any good hanging in your closet? If you feel you don't want to give them away, you can store them in case you need that size at a later date. Some people decide that if they were ever to fit into those clothes again, the styles would no longer be what they would choose to wear, so they get rid of them. Sometimes people worry about the financial expense involved in giving clothes away. They convince themselves that if only they could lose weight, the clothes would fit and they could save money. But the truth is the clothes don't fit you right now and you need something to wear.

Allowing yourself to fill your closet with clothes that fit you and support your sense of self and style is freeing and exciting. Take time to think about how you want to express yourself. Have you always worn black because it is supposed to make you look thinner? Are there other colors you want to wear instead? Purple, perhaps, or shades of pink? Or do you love black, and want to think about buying that special black dress or those flowing black pants? As you feel ready, fill your closet in a way that supports you in the same way you have stocked your kitchen with foods that you love.

ACTIVITY: Cleaning Out Your Closet

When you feel ready, clean out your closet.

- Decide what clothes currently fit you, and of those clothes, which ones you really like.

- Clear out clothes hanging in your closet that are either too big or too small. Give them away or store them.
- Begin building a wardrobe that fits your size and style.
- Consider whether you prefer to shop alone or with someone.
- Discover how you like to shop (e.g., department store, small boutique, catalogs).

"I base my fashion sense on what doesn't itch."
—Gilda Radner

LESSON #33

Let go of your scale as a way to measure yourself. It's an external means of judging, and it's likely to put you at risk for overeating.

Scales are the cornerstone of diet programs. Weekly weigh-ins tell you whether you are a "success" or "failure." If you're like most dieters, you weigh yourself much more frequently than once a week. Many people weigh themselves daily or even numerous times a day. It's not uncommon to move the scale around, take off your jewelry and clothes, and make sure you go to the bathroom before getting on the scale, all in hopes of getting a "better" reading.

There is a good chance you can tell what is happening with your weight just by the feel of your body or by the way that your clothes fit. But in a sense, what you weigh isn't really the issue. Our culture uses weight as a means of judging all kinds of things about you. When you use the scale to decide how you are doing, you buy into the notion that your weight equals your physical health and determines your self-worth. Whether you are going to have a good day or a bad day all depends on a number. You are giving a tiny box a huge amount of power!

The problem with the scale doesn't end there. Let's

say you're dieting and think you've lost weight. You get on the scale, and it confirms that, indeed, you've lost several pounds. Now what? Most dieters can relate to the experience of feeling that they deserve a reward. After all, you deprived yourself for some time in order to lose weight. Shouldn't you get to eat something you love after all that hard work?

Now let's say that you get on the scale and find that you gained weight. How do you feel? Perhaps you notice emotions such as depression, anger, hopelessness, or anxiety. These feelings also put you at risk of overeating because dieters frequently use food to soothe themselves when they experience uncomfortable feelings. So again, the scale—which was supposed to motivate you to eat less—actually increases the likelihood that you will turn to food when you're not physically hungry.

If the scale triggers overeating whether the numbers go up or down, should you ever weigh yourself? The answer is that it's best to get rid of your scale when you feel ready to do so. This isn't a means of going into denial about your weight but rather is a way of creating an environment of acceptance for yourself that will allow you to do the work of developing attuned eating skills and to let go of the negative judgments represented by the scale.

There are times when it's medically necessary to be weighed. Your weight is important to your doctor for proper medication doses or because sudden changes might indicate illness. However, there is really no reason for your doctor to weigh you when you are there for symptoms such as the flu or a sprained wrist.

Letting go of the scale may seem scary at first. It's been a lifelong companion that you relied on to keep track of yourself. Experience what it feels like to live without an external measure of your success. Instead, check in with yourself regularly from the inside to evaluate where you are on your journey. Numbers on a scale can never give you that kind of information.

ACTIVITY: Up, Up, and A-Weigh

Put your scale away, or throw it away. Keep track of how you experience your body without relying on the scale.

- Have you been eating when you are hungry, what you are hungry for, and stopping when full?
- Do your clothes feel comfortable, too big, or too small?
- Does your body feel energized or tired?

These markers can give you important information about how your body is functioning, and what changes, if any, should be addressed.

"Not everything that can be counted counts, and not everything that counts can be counted."
—Albert Einstein

LESSON #34

Live in the present. When you put off goals and activities until you lose weight, you miss out on the pleasures of life you are entitled to experience at any size.

"When I get thin, I will…" Does this phrase sound familiar to you? Dieters frequently put off important goals, believing that they must lose weight first. You might be waiting to buy a bathing suit, take an exercise class, or start dating. Whatever you are waiting for, the time to take action is *now*.

Your perceptions of how others see you and how you see yourself are preventing you from doing the things you want. Let's say that you've been wanting to take an exercise class, but not until you lose weight because you feel ashamed of your body. Begin to think about ways you might achieve your goal that would feel comfortable to you at your current size. Finding a class that caters to a diverse group of women may provide the comfort and safety you need to start moving. Or you might exercise with a tape in the privacy of your home. Maybe walking around your neighborhood feels comfortable. If your budget allows, you might work with a personal trainer who will focus on fitness rather than weight loss. The point is to let go of the idea that you must lose weight in order to start doing something that's important to you. Instead, think about how you can begin to live the life you want *right now.*

Although we used the example of exercise, this type of brainstorming can apply to all sorts of areas of your life, such as traveling, buying new clothes, or learning how to dance. Sometimes people find that there is something they thought they would do if they were thinner, but when they really explore it, the idea is no longer appealing. For example, one diet survivor told us that if she were thin, she would wear a miniskirt. Yet when she thought this through and imagined herself wearing one, she realized she would be uncomfortable exposing so much of herself, no matter what her size. This is in contrast to another diet survivor who loved the water but hadn't gone swimming in years because of her shame about wearing a bathing suit. Once she realized how painful it felt to deprive herself of an activity she loved so much, she found a bathing suit that fit and decided to wear a long skirt over it when she came out of the pool.

There are other kinds of goals that people frequently tie to weight loss. Dieters often believe that if they lose weight, they'll have increased self-esteem, feel more confident, or start dating because they'll have an easier time with intimacy. These types of goals often reflect deeper issues that need to be addressed. For example, one diet survivor insisted that once she lost weight, her relationship with her husband would improve. She did, in fact lose weight, but to her disappointment, her marriage did not improve and the couple divorced.

There is another aspect to this belief that can potentially cause a problematic situation for diet survivors. Let's say that you think that when you become thin, you'll be able to start dating. Now, let's say that through the process of attuned eating, your body naturally stabilizes at a smaller size. You set out to meet a potential partner. Yet despite your best efforts, you just cannot sustain an intimate relationship. What's happening?

Many people hook their psychological issues onto their weight. This means that they decide that their size is creating the problem, rather than looking more deeply into why they're struggling with certain issues. If this is true for you, in one way this belief gives you a sense of control. After all, if your weight is the problem and you lose the weight, your difficulties will be solved. This allows you to live with the fantasy that being thin is the magic cure, and it keeps you from having to face whatever is truly bothering you. However, if you count on weight loss to fix your problems and then find that the same problems persist even if you do lose weight, you're likely to feel an increase in mouth hunger and turn back to food to soothe your anxiety. Overeating ensures the pounds will return, leaving you again with the magical hope that becoming thin will solve life's issues. Dealing with whatever bothers you in the present and unhooking these problems from weight can only improve the quality of your life.

When you live in the present, you will need to unhook your psychological issues from your weight. This means, for example, looking into why your self-esteem is low or why you have trouble forming relationships. The benefits of taking these steps are that you can begin to address your problems now and find real solutions. Furthermore, if you do find that your body becomes thinner in response to your new way of eating, you won't get scared.

Stop waiting! Are you satisfied with the way your life is going? Are you missing out on pleasures because you don't feel entitled to do certain things at your current body size? You deserve better!

ACTIVITY: There's No Time Like the Present

Make a list of at least five things you would like in your life but have put on hold until you lose weight:

_____

_____

_____

_____

_____

Review your list and pick at least one thing you can begin today. On the lines below, write down why you would like to add this to your life, and how you can make that dream a reality.

_____

_____

_____

_____

_____

"You must live in the present, launch yourself on every wave, find your eternity in each moment."
—Henry David Thoreau

LESSON #35

Accepting your body allows you to take good care of yourself no matter what your size.

As a diet survivor, there's a good chance that you view your body as a battleground. You see fat as your enemy and have devoted much time, energy, and money trying to change your body. This attitude of self-hatred leads many people to disregard the needs of their body. Yet no matter what your size, it is essential to your well-being that you believe your body is worth taking care of.

Some diet survivors detach themselves from their bodies as a way of coping with their weight. In a sense, their size feels so upsetting to them that they disconnect their minds from the experiences of their bodies. You might notice that when you think about yourself, you picture only your head, without the rest of your body. Or you might find it distressing to think about someone touching you or you insist that the lights are off when you have sex. You might neglect signs of a physical problem that requires medical attention. These are attempts to negate the existence of your body because it feels unacceptable to you. Yet this disconnection interferes with basic self-care.

You may fear that if you accept your body at its current size, you will become complacent and never lose weight.

However, acceptance doesn't say anything about where your body will naturally stabilize once you eat in accordance with your physical hunger. The more nurturing you can be toward your body, the better able you will be to find your natural weight.

Develop a compassionate stance toward yourself, which includes the way you treat your body. You are a valuable person, and it's important that you accept yourself exactly where you are at this point. This doesn't mean that you need to pretend to love your appearance if, in fact, you do not. This is the body you inhabit and, large or small, it has needs that cannot be separated from you as a whole person. When you detach from your body and view it as your enemy, you cannot adequately meet your needs. When you accept your body as it is right now and acknowledge that you deserve to take care of yourself, you're in a stronger position to meet these needs. Think of it as a positive cycle: the more you accept yourself, the greater your ability to meet the needs of your body. And the better job you do of meeting these needs, the more connected you'll feel with your body, leading to even greater acceptance. This is a win-win situation! Your body is not your enemy. Make peace!

ACTIVITY: A Letter to Myself

Write a letter to a part of your body that elicits negative

feelings. After completing this letter, have that body part write back.

Example:

Dear Upper Arms,

I thought it was time for you to know how much I hate you. You're fat and disgusting, and I can't stand the way you jiggle. When the weather is warm, I still try to wear long sleeves because I am so embarrassed by your layers of flesh that pour out of my short-sleeved shirts. I am hot, uncomfortable, and jealous of all the people wearing summer clothes. Sometimes I look in the mirror and, with one hand, I hold your fat flesh and tighten it around my arm, wishing I could cut you off and have arms that were more acceptable. When I release the fat, I am so mad that you won't disappear that I cry. That's why I try to hide you as much as possible because looking at you makes me so depressed.

Myself

Dear Myself,

It was very hard for us to read your words. You have been too harsh with us and have given no thought to the positive things we do for you. We allow you to hold your arms out to those you love and embrace them. We held your babies for you and rocked them in the middle of the night. You used to love to swim, and we matched you stroke for stroke. Day in and day out, we help you with all of your work and chores.

Don't you think we would like to enjoy the sun and the breeze on a warm afternoon? It is hot, itchy, and uncomfortable to be covered up when we long for the fresh air. There are some people who have lost the use of their arms: people who are paralyzed or have had an arm amputated. We may not fit the cultural view of what the perfect arms should look like—thin with hard muscles—but right now, we're the arms you have. Can we please be friends? We would like to wrap ourselves around you and give you a great big hug.

Reaching out to you,
Upper Arms

_____

_____

_____

_____

_____

_____

_____

_____

_____

_____

_____

_____

_____

_____

_____
_____
_____
_____
_____
_____
_____
_____
_____
_____
_____
_____
_____
_____
_____
_____
_____
_____
_____
_____
_____
_____
_____
_____

"Self-love depressed becomes self-loathing."
—Sally Kempton

LESSON #36

Connect positively with your body as much as possible. Notice the pleasure you can experience.

As a diet survivor, you're familiar with negative body thoughts that make you feel bad. However, chances are that there are moments when you have an experience with your body that actually feels good. How much attention do you pay to these positive body thoughts?

In the lessons on eating, we emphasized the importance of collecting physical hunger experiences whenever possible, despite the fact that your mouth hunger eating might have been more frequent. This enabled you to slowly build a bank account of good caretaking, which helped you begin to see your way out of overeating. Likewise, this is an important strategy to use with your body experiences. As you work toward building a stronger body image, actively noticing that you have pleasurable feelings with the body you have now will help you understand that it's *not* an objective fact that your body is unlovable. Rather, you *can* move in the direction of developing an attitude of care and acceptance of yourself.

For example, let's say you've just stepped out of the shower and you decide to put a special lotion on your body. You notice how good it feels to rub on the lotion and how soft your skin feels. Enjoy these sensations! Perhaps you've just bought a new outfit to wear to a special occasion. You look in the mirror and think what a beautiful color it is on you, how it complements your eyes and skin tone. Again, take in the positive feeling.

A massage allows your body to feel relaxed, while a compliment about your hairstyle from a friend leaves you feeling pleased. A bike ride lets you feel the strength of your body, while yoga leaves you feeling flexible and connected to yourself. All of these examples build the notion that you can have positive thoughts about your body *at your current size.*

As you collect these positive body thoughts, notice whether you actively stop yourself from enjoying them. For example, do you ever ask, "How could I possibly feel so good about myself when I feel so fat?" The answer is that you are entitled to have good feelings about your body no matter what your shape and size. Negative body thoughts will most likely return, but for the moment, try to stay present and allow yourself the pleasurable experience.

The relationship you have with your body is always in a state of flux. However, you can actively make decisions about how to care for your body, such as in the way you dress, move, and touch it. Your goal is to notice times when you have good experiences in your body. When you do, play them up to yourself by saying, "Wow, this is terrific. I feel really good right now." This will help you counteract those other moments when you feel overcome by negative body thoughts and will help you develop a more loving relationship with your body.

ACTIVITY: Collecting Positive Body Experiences

Supplies:
- A jar or old shoe box (feel free to decorate)
- 3x5 note cards (at least ten) cut in half
- Pen

For the next few weeks, stay mindful of your positive body experiences. Fill out a note card describing your experiences. What were you doing? How did you feel? Describe what you liked about the experience. After you have finished, drop it in your jar or box. Soon you'll have a collection of positive body experiences. Occasionally pull out a card to read. Continue to find new ways to experience the pleasure of your body.

"Pleasure is Nature's test, her sign of approval."
—*Oscar Wilde*

LESSON #37

As you feel stronger about your own body image, it will become easier to reject the negative messages of others.

Every day you are bombarded with messages about the desirability of losing weight. Until now, those messages matched your own beliefs about the importance of becoming thinner. As you work on acceptance, you are challenging and changing the way you think about your size. You're learning that you can be healthy and feel attractive, even if your body doesn't conform to the cultural ideal.

As you feel stronger, it will become easier for you to reject the messages of the media and other people in your life. When a comment or ad is directed at you, bounce it right back to its source. Keep in mind the idea that when people make negative statements about weight, they are projecting their own feelings onto you. After all, the people in your life are equally susceptible to all of the messages about thinness and dieting as you have been. You have a choice to make. You can take in what is being said and feel bad about yourself, or you can reject the message and refuse to internalize the comment. You empower yourself when you make the choice not to take in the negative messages of the culture in whatever form they arrive.

There may be times when you feel stronger than others. Diet survivors often struggle when ads for new diets hit the airwaves. It can feel difficult to resist a new promise and not worry about your size when everyone else is jumping on the diet bandwagon. Do your best to avoid weight-loss commercials and ads. Remind yourself that the majority of people who start these plans will soon be off their diets.

You may find that you feel strongly about your decision not to diet when you're by yourself, but as soon as you're around others, it becomes harder to ignore the negative messages about weight. It can feel painful when the people you love, and who love you, tell you that you're not okay the way you are. Criticism about your body size or food choices might make you feel doubtful about yourself or might make you feel angry. In either case, by taking in the reactions and feelings of others, you weaken your own commitment to being a diet survivor journeying toward greater physical and psychological well-being.

Consider having a discussion with the people whose comments affect you and letting them know about the changes you're making in your life. Some people will be receptive to hearing and understanding what you're trying to do, and some won't. The truth is that ideas about weight loss are so entrenched in our culture that many people just can't believe there is another point of view.

Your family and friends might have their own issues about body size and may be actively dieting. Your ideas about becoming an attuned eater and developing a stance of acceptance may feel threatening to them. If this is the case, see if you can reach a truce, and agree to disagree. Tell them that you know they want to help you but that you are acting in a manner that you believe is in your best interest. If they cannot fully support you, ask them if they can at least refrain from making comments about your weight and eating.

Some diet survivors find themselves in relationships where a significant person won't stop berating them about weight. In this case, it can be very difficult to constantly resist negative remarks. Sometimes another person's comments are so hurtful that they qualify as verbal abuse. If someone is frequently calling you names or making fun of you because of your body size, that is *not* okay. No matter how hard you work on becoming stronger, these types of assaults weaken you and make it virtually impossible to resist taking in the negative messages. If you are in this situation, consider the overall quality of the relationship. Chances are there are other areas of dysfunction that indicate an unhealthy relationship. Don't buy into the idea that your weight is the cause of these problems and that once you lose weight, everything will be all right. If you cannot figure out how to change the dynamics of the relationship on your own, consider seeking professional help, preferably with a person who is already familiar with the concept of a non-diet approach.

The accumulation of attuned eating experiences and the work of building self-acceptance give you more and more positive feelings about yourself, which help you feel stronger on the inside. This strength allows you to stop taking in messages that promote dieting and weight loss as the avenue to physiological and psychological well-being. Instead, your new experiences and knowledge give you the power to reject these messages. Always remember that when you take in what others tell you, you give them power. Find your own strength.

ACTIVITY: Be Like Teflon, and Don't Let It Stick

You've heard the advertising boast "Nothing sticks to Teflon." Well, we want you to become like that nonstick pan. When you hear or see negative messages, either from the culture at large or a significant other, imagine the comments sliding right off you. If you find certain messages sticking despite your best efforts, write them down. Messages that seem to stick:

_____

_____

_____

As you read over these messages, see if you can come up with a response that reinforces a stance of acceptance.

_____

_____

_____

"My mother's menu consisted of two choices: Take it or leave it."
—Buddy Hackett

LESSON #38

Negative body thoughts are often a way of talking to yourself about other issues in your life that bother you. Learn to decode these messages.

Have you ever wondered why sometimes you feel fine in your body and at other times you're plagued with negative thoughts? We have discussed at length the reasons that make it so hard to feel good about yourself in this culture. However, there are psychological factors that also affect the way you feel about your body at a particular moment.

In the lessons on eating, we explained that sometimes you might reach for food because an emotion is too uncomfortable to experience. The reach for food helps you move away from whatever is really bothering you. You translate your problem into one of food and weight rather than acknowledging that you have a problem managing uncomfortable feelings. Likewise, there are times that you might elicit a negative body thought to distance yourself from a particular feeling and make yourself believe that it's a problem with your size. However, as Hirschmann and Munter discuss in *When Women Stop Hating Their Bodies,* you are actually translating an uncomfortable feeling into a negative body thought.

Imagine you've been invited to a party. As you put on

your outfit, all sorts of negative thoughts come to mind. You know that a colleague from work will also be there, and lately, you've had the feeling that he's flirting with you. Even though your boyfriend or spouse will be with you and you have no intention of acting on the coworker's interest, deep down you realize that you feel some attraction to him. This leaves you feeling extremely uncomfortable. As you look in the mirror you find yourself thinking that your thighs look disgusting and wonder how you can possibly attend.

Can you see how this discomfort was placed onto your body? You called your thighs disgusting when what really disgusts you is the fact that you feel attracted to someone other than your significant other. You translated this underlying feeling into the actual words you used to criticize your body, which allowed you to distance yourself from the original emotion. The negative body thoughts that you directed toward yourself allowed you to consider not going to the party, thereby helping you avoid the situation that led to the uncomfortable feeling in the first place.

Learning to decode your negative body thoughts can give you important information about yourself. It can also help you end the yelling about your size when you understand that you're using your body and the accepted language of the culture to communicate something important. Start by looking at the words you use to describe yourself. There are many ways to talk to yourself about your body, yet you choose particular, specific adjectives. These words are significant.

Next, ask yourself what aspect of your personality or situation in life the words describe. For example, if you say that your stomach "sticks out," think about what else sticks out about you. If you describe yourself as "too big," ask yourself if there is there anything else in your life that feels too big right now. You may be surprised how closely the words you use reflect a circumstance of your life.

One diet survivor stated she had a "big behind." Much of the time she felt okay with her body, and she became curious about why these thoughts popped up from time to time. As she looked at the words, she had an association. She explained that she was the oldest of five children. Her mother was quite depressed during her childhood, and therefore much of the responsibility for her siblings fell to her. She remembered walking down the street to take all of her brothers and sisters home, and as they followed her she felt that there was a "big behind." In other words, all of this big responsibility was following right behind her. She used this understanding to be compassionate with herself about how hard it was to have to be the adult in her home when she was still a child. Furthermore, whenever that negative body thought came to mind, she could now remind herself that it wasn't really about her body. Rather, thinking about her "big behind" meant that something had triggered her feelings about her childhood. This put her in a position to think about and understand what was really bothering her.

Decoding your negative body thoughts is a skill that takes practice. You may protest that the words you use to berate yourself have no meaning. You might say that the truth is that you are fat and that the thoughts you have are in direct response to your size. We encourage you to look again and look a little deeper. While it's true that there is much language in our culture that teaches you to criticize your body, you have also developed a language to disguise certain feelings. There's a reason that your negative body thoughts occur at certain times and that you pick particular words to describe yourself.

Another way to learn more about the psychological meaning of your negative body thoughts is to ask yourself what you might be thinking about at a particular moment if you were not having that negative thought. When it comes to food, you've learned to ask yourself, "I'm reaching for food but I'm not hungry. I wonder what I might think about or feel if I didn't eat right now?" You can do the same with your negative thoughts as you ask, "I'm yelling at myself about my body. I wonder what would be on my mind right now if I weren't criticizing myself?" If you can trace your way back to whatever thoughts and feelings preceded the negative thoughts, you might learn something important about the kinds of emotions that trigger your discomfort.

Think of yourself as a detective. In addition to the work you are already doing to build a more positive body image and actively end the self-criticism of yourself, try to uncover the meaning of the negative body thoughts that linger. The words you use and the context in which you use them do mean something. Decoding your negative thoughts helps you directly face other issues in your life that bother you. It also helps you to move in the direction of acceptance as you increasingly understand that the words you use to talk to yourself about your body are not objective facts. Rather, you're using the talk of body hatred, sanctioned by our culture, to disguise feelings that are unacceptable to you.

ACTIVITY : Decoding Negative Body Thoughts

Write down the most common negative body thought that you have.

_____

_____

_____

Next, circle the adjective that you use to describe your body. Below, try to uncover what this code word might really be about. Relax and brainstorm away. Think of what else in your life you would use that particular word for, and then see if there is a connection.

_____

_____

_____

Finally, write down your ideas about what your negative body thought might really be about.

_____

_____

_____

> *"Hear the meaning within the word."*
> *—William Shakespeare*

LESSON #39

Bodies change throughout the life cycle. Acceptance means finding comfort with yourself and appreciating the full capacities of your body at any age and size.

The human body changes dramatically throughout the life cycle. The infant grows into an active child, who then undergoes the changes of puberty. The young adult woman experiences changes during pregnancy and breast-feeding. The middle-aged body matures and continues to transform. All of these changes are natural and not easily altered. Yet at the same time, we tend to hold on to a mental image of ourselves at a particular body size and view that as our natural weight. Usually, we choose a body image that most closely conforms to the standards of the culture. Currently, the most culturally desirable body image is young and thin. Chances are that wherever you were closest to this ideal is where you consider your natural body weight to be.

While you might think about body size in terms of what our culture considers attractive, from an evolutionary point of view our bodies are oblivious to these ideals. You cannot easily override your body's physiology; when you try to do so, your efforts are likely to backfire. For example, during puberty the female body adds fat cells to the hips, stomach, thighs, and breasts to prepare for pregnancy, thereby ensuring survival of the human species. When a girl responds to these changes by dieting, her body goes on high alert. The body assumes it is a time of famine. In response, *even more fat cells are created, and they are larger than they would have been under natural circumstances.* When she goes off the diet, her body becomes even more efficient at storing fat to make sure she'll have enough to reproduce even if there is another "famine." Her dieting has had the opposite effect of what was intended, and this individual will probably end up at a higher weight than where she was naturally meant to be. Studies done on adolescents who diet in high school find that they end up larger than their non-dieting counterparts.

During pregnancy and lactation, the female body shifts significantly yet again. Many women find weight issues predominant during these times. For some, pregnancy becomes a license to remove former restrictions and eat anything regardless of hunger, while others restrict their food intake in order to control their weight gain. For some, breast-feeding becomes the newest weight-loss method to try to quickly get rid of the added pounds from pregnancy. In these examples, the natural wonders of the body are sacrificed to focus on weight issues.

Menopause also brings changes to female physiology as fat cells naturally increase in order to ease the transition.

According to nutritionist Debra Waterhouse, the more you fight this increase in fat cells by dieting, the more powerful your menopausal fat cells become, guaranteeing a greater weight gain. Again, the individual's attempt to change her powerful physiology works against her as attempts to become thinner only strengthen the determination of her fat cells.

Most dieters want to return to and maintain the lowest weight they reached in the past. You might assume that this is your ideal body weight and believe that once you get back there, you will be satisfied. In a culture that values youth, part of the issue is that we tend to associate the "thinner body" with a "younger body." Therefore, the idea of getting back to a thinner you is a way of postponing feelings you might have about getting older. Directly confronting, or at least exploring your feelings about aging, can free up a tremendous amount of energy and allow you to focus on the important tasks at hand in your current life stage. The other part of the issue is the myth that it's possible to return to the weight of a previous phase in your life. Very few people look the way they did in high school. Our bodies really do change in shape and size over the years as the result of numerous factors.

Consider changing your view of the cycle of your body. Think about valuing its capacities at every stage. Instead of thinking about one body size as better than another, consider how amazing it is that your body knows just what to do to get you through life. Then, enjoy each stage without judging the changes in your body that naturally occur. They aren't better or worse, just different—and always worth appreciating.

ACTIVITY: The Beauty of Each Season

You are the same person as you were before, yet you are constantly changing. This is the way of nature: the flower grows from seed to bud to blossom and then withers; the seasons move from spring to summer to fall to winter. Each stage holds its own wonder and beauty.

Write down at least two thoughts that capture the wonder of the life cycle at each phase. Use either full sentences or list adjectives to convey your feelings. Try to connect with your body, mind, and spirit. Stay away from commenting on weight, and focus instead on capturing your place within the natural order of things.

Childhood

_____

_____

_____

Teens

_____

_____

_____

Early Adulthood

_____

_____

_____

Middle Age

_____

_____

_____

Later Years

_____

_____

_____

*"No man ever steps in the same river twice; for it's not the same
river and he's not the same man."*
—Heracleitus

LESSON #40

The words thin and fat are limiting. Learn to find other adjectives to describe your body.

Take a moment to think about how you view your body. If you are reading this book, you probably do not see yourself as thin. Therefore, do you consider yourself to be fat? There is a good chance that no matter what your size, you find yourself "feeling fat" much of the time, and this feeling is fraught with negative connotations. However, thin and fat are just descriptions of size rather than valid indicators of people's worth or behavior.

Language is the means we have to transfer our internal thoughts, beliefs, and feelings to ourselves and others. The word thin is currently the most common adjective in our language used to describe what is considered to be the desirable body type in our culture. At this point in our history, the definition of thin is extremely stringent; for most people, being thin enough means having no evidence of fat on the body. Yet this ideal is nearly impossible. Since there are no other words commonly used to describe the range between the thinnest of human beings to the largest, many diet survivors immediately jump to the conclusion that if they are not thin, they must be fat. Of course, we do not mean to imply in any way that fat is "bad" or thin is "good"; people naturally come in different shapes and sizes. Rather, we want to emphasize the narrow definition placed on body size that is long on value judgment and short on true descriptiveness.

What words exist in our language to describe the natural range of body sizes? Some of the ones we can think of, such as pudgy, plump, husky, or chubby, have negative connotations. The word average is sometimes used, but lacks much imagination or desirability. Euphemisms such as big-boned or voluptuous also fail to offer a truly positive identity to attach to body size. Perhaps the real problem is that our body image is too broad of a concept to count on a single word to capture ourselves. Perhaps we have, as a culture, overloaded the word *thin* with too much meaning so that people are striving to diminish themselves in order to fit into a meaningless category. Any diet survivor who has used a personal ad or online dating service, in which you must give a one word description of your body size in order to participate, knows how difficult and shaming this task can be.

We do not have a solution to this problem of semantics, but we do want to alert you to it. There is a whole natural range of body sizes, and the words *thin* and *fat* are insufficient to capture the diversity of human beings. Try to be more creative in how you assign a description of your body to yourself. If we looked at a continuum, some of you would fall into the thinner range and some of you would fall into the fatter range. Yet your body is so much more than a word. Expand the way you use language to describe your body to yourself and others. Embrace the wholeness of yourself.

ACTIVITY : I Am...

Below is a list of adjectives that describe a person's body. Circle the ones that apply to you:

Flexible	Soft	Relaxed
Strong	Supple	Spry
Curvy	Graceful	Hardy
Muscular	Poised	Robust
Sturdy	Balanced	Vigorous
Agile	Healthy	Dynamic
		Energetic

Did you notice that all of these words have positive connotations?

"Much of what we see depends on what we are looking for."
—Phil Calloway

LESSON #41

It's natural to continue to want to lose weight, no matter how hard you work on acceptance. Recognize that when weight loss occurs, it's a side effect of normalizing your relationship with food, rather than the main goal.

We hope that as a result of your hard work you've developed a more positive relationship with your body. This doesn't mean that you'll never have moments when you still experience negative body thoughts. However, you're likely to notice a decrease in the frequency and intensity of these thoughts. You have a greater understanding that your negative body thoughts are the result of faulty messages that you have internalized rather than objective facts about your inherent beauty, health, and self-worth. You also have the tools to explore any underlying psychological meaning contained in your self-criticism.

The goal of self-acceptance is to feel good about yourself at any size. Yet, because of the intense pressures in our culture to become thinner, it's understandable that you may continue to hope that you'll lose weight as the result of this process. There is nothing wrong with acknowledging this feeling. After all, part of your journey is being able to notice feelings without using food to make them go away.

Most people who learn about this approach believe that they'll lose weight as a result of their work. This is because they know that they're currently eating more food than their bodies need as the result of the diet/binge cycle; they assume that once they normalize their eating, they'll eat less. You can expect to stabilize at your natural size as the result of this process, and for some of you that will be at a lower weight. However, unlike diet programs in which weight loss occurs quickly—followed by regaining the weight—diet survivors who lose weight with this approach do so over a longer period of time.

If you begin practicing eating as an attuned eater after you have just been on a diet, chances are you will initially regain some weight as your body responds to the recent deprivation. You must remember that after any period of dieting, 95 to 98 percent of people will regain the weight. As your body becomes accustomed to a more reliable way of eating, it will adjust accordingly.

If you have been restricting for most of your life and trying to weigh less than your body was meant to weigh, you might find your body settles at a higher range than you had been struggling to maintain. If, in the past, you have been eating less from stomach hunger and more from mouth hunger, or if you have dieted your way up to a higher weight than what is natural for you, your weight may settle at a lower range.

If and when weight loss occurs, it's important to think of it as a side effect of the work you are doing. Throughout this process, you are making yourself physically and emotionally healthier by normalizing your relationship with food, dealing directly with your feelings, taking care of your physical health, moving your body, and improving your self-esteem through acceptance. This is the focus of your work. None of this is about weight loss. So, if it happens, it's merely an adjustment that your body is making to your new way of living.

Here's why this attitude is so important. If you continue to feel that losing weight is the most important part of this process, you set yourself up to overeat. Let's say you notice that you've been eating mostly out of stomach hunger and now your clothes are looser. You get excited! You tell yourself this is great—this approach is really working. But then the next time you are physically hungry for cookies, you have second thoughts. After all, you've started to lose weight. And you still remember the calorie count of cookies. So you decide not to eat them. But sooner or later you feel deprived (of course). Even if you do allow yourself to eat them in the moment, just the thought that you "shouldn't" eat them and might take them away again is enough to cause a diet survivor to feel deprived. Eventually you make up for that deprivation by overeating the very cookies that you avoided or by overeating something else. Or you decide that from now on, you'll only eat when you're physically hungry. You try to control your emotional hunger, rather than gently moving in the direction of stomach hunger. As the result of these changes, you notice an overall increase in your overeating. Before you know it, your clothes are tight again.

The paradox of this process is that the less you care about losing weight, the more likely you are to lose it. You cannot trick yourself into this stance, so keep working on acceptance. Think of the idea that while you are on this path, your weight is none of your business. In our experience, by the time diet survivors do lose weight through this approach, it's no longer such a big deal. Instead, they already feel quite comfortable with themselves and are pleased with the many positive changes they've made in their lives. The weight loss is a reflection of these changes, not the main event. This doesn't mean that if you do lose weight, you cannot feel pleased. Perhaps you notice that your thighs no longer rub together, and the relief from the chafing is welcome. Or you might find that it is easier to buy clothes, which feels good. Yet your excitement stays in proportion to how weight loss fits into your life, rather than becoming an indicator of your success.

It's also important to keep in mind that not everyone will lose weight with this process. As discussed in previous lessons, many factors determine your natural size. You have control over some aspects of your life but not others. You cannot fight genetics. You cannot undo years of yo-yo dieting. The effects of illnesses or medications may also be beyond your control. Acceptance enables you to find a place of peace with yourself, and you deserve that. Most diet survivors find that their weight stabilizes over time, which means that they no longer have the constant ups and downs in their size. As a result, they don't need to have different sizes of clothes or wonder from season to season what will fit them. They accept—or work toward accepting—that they have achieved their natural weight. They're sustained by the relief they get when they aren't preoccupied by food and from the better body image they're building. You too can experience these positive feelings.

ACTIVITY: A Booster Shot to Remember the Goal

Here's a list of the goals that are part of the path you're on. Give an example of how each goal has been manifested on your journey to remind yourself of the wonderful work you're doing. Celebrate the many ways you're enriching your life!

Normalizing my eating has

_____

_____

_____

Becoming more compassionate with myself has

_____

_____

_____

Dealing with my feelings directly has

_____

_____

_____

Practicing acceptance has

_____

_____

_____

"Every day you may make progress. Every step may be fruitful.
Yet there will stretch out before you an ever-lengthening, ever-
ascending, ever-improving path. You know you will never get
to the end of the journey. But this, so far from discouraging,
only adds to the joy and glory of the climb."
—*Winston Churchill*

LESSON #42

Be aware of any mixed feelings you might have about weight loss.

Almost every diet survivor who strives to normalize her relationship with food hopes that one of the outcomes will include weight loss. Yet as much as people say they want to lose weight, sometimes they actually have mixed feelings about becoming thinner. It's important to identify any conflicting emotions you have regarding weight loss so that if your body naturally becomes thinner as a result of this approach, you'll feel comfortable with these changes. Remember, the goal of acceptance is to allow your body to stabilize at its natural size. We wouldn't want you to end up at an artificially high weight any more than we would want you to try to maintain a weight that is unnaturally low for you.

One diet survivor realized that when she imagined losing weight, she thought that people would expect more of her. In her mind, she assumed she would have more energy. Yet she already felt overloaded, and the thought of having to do even more was enough to overwhelm her. Therefore, at an unconscious level, staying heavier felt safer. As she became aware of these feelings, she was able to unhook her size from the amount of commitments she made. It was only by becoming aware of the way she associated thinness with an increased activity level that she was able to resolve this conflict.

Another diet survivor identified a connection between weight loss and a fear that went back to her difficult childhood. As a survivor of sexual abuse, she viewed her weight as a means of protecting herself. When she began to lose weight as a natural part of normalizing her eating, she discovered a strong need to use her fat as a boundary between herself and the world. As she noticed herself getting thinner, she had a sudden increase in overeating. As she reflected on what was happening, she realized that weight loss frightened her and made her feel more vulnerable to being abused. Her task was to see herself as an adult who has resources to protect herself from unwanted intrusion and to feel that she could adequately set boundaries. Only when she felt able to separate her experience as a child from her capabilities as an adult was she able to allow herself to resume her normal eating.

One diet survivor believed that he would begin dating once he became thin yet realized that he was frightened of intimacy and scared to begin the process. He worked on the idea that even if he lost weight, he didn't need to start dating if he didn't feel ready. At the same time, he decided to tackle his concerns about relationships at his current size.

The key is for you to unhook body size from whatever issues cause concern. You've spent years blaming your body size for some problems and counting on becoming thin to solve others. You've invested all sorts of meaning into your weight, and you might not even be aware that you've done so! While you were imagining all the positive outcomes you hoped to receive as the result of becoming thinner, you may have skipped over some of the fears you also associate with weight loss. Now is the time to check in with yourself so that if weight loss does occur, it can take place without mixed feelings.

How will you know if you have mixed feelings about weight loss? The most common way that attuned eaters discover their ambivalence is when an initial weight loss is followed by a puzzling increase in mouth hunger. If this happens for you, reflect on whether there is anything about losing weight that feels uncomfortable.

If you do find that there is something about becoming thinner that increases your anxiety, start working on this situation. Think about what meaning you have attached to weight loss and start unhooking the idea of becoming thinner from other factors in your life.

ACTIVITY: A Visualization to Ease Ambivalence

After reading the instructions, close your eyes and imagine these scenarios. Then reflect on the questions.

- Imagine that you are thinner and you into walk into a party. How do you feel as you enter the room? What are you thinking and feeling? Where do you place yourself at the party? Are you standing alone, with one or two people, or in a crowd? How would you describe your experience at the party? As good as being thin may feel, can you identify any uncomfortable feelings?

- Imagine yourself entering this same party at a heavier weight. How do you feel as you enter the room? What are you thinking and feeling? Where do you place yourself at the party? Are you standing alone, with one or two people, or in a crowd? How would you describe your experience at the party? As difficult as being heavier may feel, can you identify how this body size helps you in any way?

By identifying psychological issues that might have become hooked onto weight, you're in a better position to allow your body to find and relax into its natural weight.

> *"Me, ambivalent? Well, yes and no."*
> *—Unknown*

LESSON #43

Decide how you want to respond to compliments about weight loss, should it occur.

You may wonder what possibly could be the problem with receiving compliments for weight loss. After all, this is probably what you are hoping for. However, diet survivors who take this journey usually find that their reactions to these compliments change significantly over time. This occurs because they understand weight loss is a side effect of this process, not the main event. When other people focus on weight loss as the sign of success, it can feel as is if these words, offered with the best of intentions, actually undermine your commitment to letting go of weight as the criteria for success. It may feel that, once again, all that matters is the number on the scale, rather than recognizing all of the substantial changes you're making in the areas of eating, acceptance, and self-care.

Many diet survivors find that when they make the expected polite response to a compliment and say thank you, they feel they've betrayed themselves by reinforcing cultural messages about thinness. Yet, some response is required when someone says, "You look great. Have you lost weight?" When you find yourself in this situation, think about what reaction feels most comfortable to you.

Sometimes people will comment that you look like you've lost weight when, in fact, there has been no change. Frequently, diet survivors feel better as the result of their work with ending dieting and taking better care of themselves. This may come through in the way you dress, carry yourself, or show more calmness or confidence in your manner. People frequently assume that if you feel better, weight loss is involved. In this situation, consider responding that what they are noticing are some changes you've recently made in your life and that you are feeling quite well, thank you very much!

If someone mentions your weight loss, and you know this to be true, there are many ways you can respond. Some diet survivors say, "You know, I no longer focus on my weight. But I am feeling very good—thank you." Others say, "I prefer not to discuss weight," while others use this as an opportunity to educate people about ending diets. In this case you might say, "I know you mean that as a compliment. But I've stopped focusing on weight loss and it's amazing. Instead, I've learned to become a normal eater. So if I've lost weight, it's just a natural part of the process for me."

Another dilemma might occur when other people in your life lose weight and expect a compliment from you. While you certainly don't want to offend them, you must also consider whether you are willing to contribute to the notion that losing weight by dieting is positive. This situation is complicated by your knowledge that odds are they'll gain the weight back. If you tell them how great they look, how will each of you feel when the weight returns? Are you comfortable with the idea that you might contribute to some of the shame they experience when the weight comes back? Will you make a comment then? There is no easy answer here, and how you respond will depend on the relationship you have with each person. However, becoming aware of these issues gives you the opportunity to think through how you want to respond to the issue of compliments so that you have a better chance of maintaining your integrity in these situations.

ACTIVITY: "You look great—have you lost weight?"

Take some time now to consider how you might choose to respond in these situations.

"Wow, you look fantastic! How much weight have you lost?"

_____

_____

_____

"I was watching you at the holiday party and saw that you hardly ate anything. You were being so good. What diet are you on?"

_____

_____

_____

"I just started a new diet. You look like you've lost some weight recently. How about we help each other stay on our diets and lose weight together by spring?"

_____

_____

_____

"You look different. Have you lost weight?"

_____

_____

_____

"Happiness is when what you think, what you say, and what you do are in harmony."
—Mahatma Gandhi

A Final Note on Acceptance

"We must be the change we wish to see in the world."
—Mahatma Gandhi

As you make these changes, it is useful to stay mindful of how your attitude of self-acceptance can affect others. After all, you are part of the culture, and your thoughts and actions can have the power to transform the people in your life. What you do, say, or model can have the ability to positively impact another potential diet survivor.

Think of a pebble being tossed into the ocean. It creates a ripple that carries further and further away from where the pebble first landed. You are that pebble and your new ways of being create those ripples. Where will they land? Who will they touch?

The culture has clear messages at this point in time about the value of thinness. But our culture is comprised of people like you. When enough people make a decision to do things differently, the culture is changed. As you continue to cultivate your own sense of self-worth and self-acceptance, you set the stage for others. You have power. Being the change you want to see is a gift you give to yourself and to the world.

6

Lessons on Self-Care

"Self-care is never a selfish act—it is simply good stewardship of the only gift I have, the gift I was put on this earth to offer others."
—Parker Palmer

LESSON #44

See your doctor on a regular basis. Learn to become an advocate for yourself.

Regular medical attention is an important aspect of self-care. Yet, many diet survivors dread seeing their doctors and may even avoid these visits completely. The idea of being weighed might fill you with anxiety, as you anticipate a long, stern lecture about the importance of losing weight. Your doctor might even recommend a specific plan, program, or nutritionist to help you shed pounds. This advice might contribute to your feelings of shame or leave you feeling helpless and hopeless because you've already tried so hard to diet. You might also find that once you leave your doctor's office, you overeat—a result of anticipating deprivation or from the anxiety created by the visit.

Given these pitfalls, what can you do? Remember that your doctor wants you to be healthy. Your doctor has taken the Hippocratic oath to "first do no harm." However, medical professionals are frequently unaware of the dangers of dieting as well as the alternatives to dieting. They've been trained to tell patients to lose weight, and they continue to do so despite the fact that there's absolutely no diet that can show positive, long-term results. In our experience, most doctors realize how difficult it is for patients to lose and maintain weight loss, but they don't know what else to offer. Hopefully, more doctors will become familiar with the research that shows that diets don't work and that weight cycling actually contributes to physical problems. Recognizing that people can improve their health at every size by becoming fit and normalizing eating will go a long way toward contributing to the physical and mental health of patients.

As you feel stronger in developing an attitude of acceptance toward yourself, you will be ready to assert your needs. Although it can be hard to question your doctor, you are entitled to have your questions answered and your requests respected.

In the lessons on acceptance, we discussed the importance of letting go of the scale. What should you do when your doctor wants to weigh you? Some diet survivors explain that they prefer not to know what they weigh and choose to get on the scale backwards. Others question whether it is really necessary to be weighed at all and often find that the staff is responsive to this request (although there are circumstances in which it is necessary to know your weight). If your doctor uses your weight to scare or shame you, speak up. Let your doctor know that you are at the office about your symptoms, not about your weight. One diet survivor reported that the lab work at her physical exam showed her to be in excellent physical health. Yet on the way out the door, her doctor told her that she really should lose some weight. She turned to him and asked why, since he had just told her how healthy she was. The doctor apologized and withdrew his recommendation.

If you do have health issues that are commonly associated with higher weights, then there is a very good chance that your doctor will recommend weight loss as part of a treatment plan. Remember that the problem with this advice is that for 95–98 percent of dieters, short-term weight loss is followed by a return to their previous weight or to an even higher weight. Furthermore, weight cycling contributes to poor health. With this information in mind, consider asking your doctor if your health problem ever exists in thinner people. The answer will inevitably be yes. Next, ask your doctor what he or she usually does in those cases, and expect to receive the same treatment. Are there medications that can help? Does exercise have an effect? Are there dietary changes (not diets) that might improve your situation? Do your best to get some recommendations other than weight loss before you walk out the door.

Part of being a diet survivor is the understanding that if you could lose weight through dieting, you would have done so by now. It is recognizing that what you weigh is not a sign of being bad or lazy. Speaking up to someone in authority takes courage. Yet ultimately you are in charge of taking care of your body and making sure that you get the treatment you need. Do your best to keep your body healthy through behaviors over which you have control, and let your doctor know that you want the best treatment possible based on factors other than body size.

ACTIVITY: What's Up, Doc?

Put a check next to the points you would like to speak up about with your doctor. Make a list to bring along to your next visit:

- Why I am giving up diets.
- Why I am focusing on health factors unrelated to weight.
- Why I don't want to be weighed at each office visit.
- Why I am interested in ways to improve my health that don't focus on weight loss.
- If you diagnose a problem, like high blood pressure, and tell me to lose weight, I would ask you to consider what you would tell a thin (or thinner) person with the same blood pressure readings and to use that as an indicator for my treatment as well.

"I told my doctor I get very tired when I go on a diet, so he gave me pep pills. Know what happened? I ate faster."
—Joe E. Lewis

LESSON #45

Fitness promotes health. As you feel ready, move your body in ways that feel comfortable to you.

Fitness helps just about everything. It can improve blood pressure, cholesterol, and diabetes. It can reduce the risk of osteoporosis and relieve a variety of aches and pains. It can increase energy, lead to mental well-being, and even extend your life. *All of these benefits take place regardless of whether any weight is lost.*

If you already have a regular exercise routine that works well for you, that's terrific. However, as a diet survivor you might have a difficult time starting or sustaining exercise. In fact, you might approach exercise like a diet. Your motivation is weight loss. You begin with the resolve that this time you'll make it work. You start out with great enthusiasm, but the day comes when you miss your work-out and you just stop. You feel guilty about not exercising, but you just can't get yourself to do it. So, you do nothing.

It can take time to break the associations between exercise, dieting, and weight loss. In order to do so, think about other reasons to take care of yourself in this way. Do you want to become more fit? Healthier? Stronger? More flexible? All of these reasons can give you the motivation to begin to move your body without focusing on weight.

There are many types of exercise. Aerobic activity, such as walking, swimming, and bike riding, improves your heart function. Anaerobic exercise, such as lifting weights, increases your muscle mass and helps reduce the risk of osteoporosis. Dance, yoga, and Pilates improve your balance, flexibility, and strength.

Think about what type of exercise you might enjoy and what would be the most comfortable setting. Do you prefer to walk on your own, or does it sound more appealing to take a yoga class? Do you like the idea of joining a health club that has lots of equipment or classes to choose from? If you do decide to go to this route, make sure you don't get caught up in their focus on weight loss as the primary reason for joining. Let them know that you are there to improve your overall physical well-being, and choose not to be weighed or measured. If, however, being in this setting fosters negative body thoughts for you, consider finding a less competitive atmosphere.

When you start to engage in physical activity, think about the amount that feels right to you. It's okay to start out slowly. Take time to build up to a level that feels good. You don't have to keep doing more and more. The key is to start moving and pay attention to how you feel. When you find pleasure in what you're doing and feel better afterward, you're much more likely to integrate activity into your life.

Some diet survivors may find themselves at the opposite end of the continuum. If you must work out for long periods of time every day in order to feel "okay," then you might have a problem with compulsive exercise. While others may admire you for your dedication to exercise, over-activity is a serious problem that can negatively affect your health. Try to cut back on your routine. If you cannot do this on your own, consult a professional.

Exercise is an important element of self-care. Allow yourself time and space to experiment with the many ways to move your body. Remember that if weight loss is your motivation to become active, it's likely to backfire. Instead, focus on the joy of movement and the knowledge that when you choose to exercise, you are choosing to take good care of yourself.

ACTIVITY: Stepping Up and Stepping Out!

Here is a list of activities you might want to consider. Put a smiley face next to the ones you'd like to try, a question mark next to the ones you might want to try, and a frown face next to the ones that hold no interest for you. Feel free to add other activities you want to try.

☐ Aerobics Class
☐ Ballet
☐ Belly Dancing
☐ Biking

- [ ] Bowling
- [ ] Dance
- [ ] Fencing
- [ ] Fitness Center
- [ ] Hiking
- [ ] Karate
- [ ] Pilates
- [ ] Rollerblading
- [ ] Running
- [ ] Racquetball
- [ ] Spinning
- [ ] Swimming
- [ ] Tai Chi
- [ ] Tennis
- [ ] Walking
- [ ] Weight Lifting
- [ ] Yoga

"My grandmother started walking five miles a day when she was sixty. She's ninety-seven today and we don't know where the hell she is."
—Ellen DeGeneres

LESSON #46

It's important to separate exercise from weight loss. If you're having trouble getting going, explore obstacles that might be getting in your way.

Often people express the wish to exercise, yet just cannot seem to do it. Are you one of those people? You may notice that you feel better when you exercise, but just can't seem to find time. You believe that there are benefits other than weight loss to moving your body, yet still do not incorporate physical activity into your life. Of course, there are some people who do not want to exercise. If this applies to you, you don't need to feel guilty. This is your life, and you're in charge of how you will take care of yourself. You're entitled to decide that exercise isn't one of the things you want to do at this point in time. However, if you are someone who wants to exercise, try to understand the obstacles that stand in your way.

Start with the most concrete possibilities. Is there a time of day you can carve out for exercise? Do you know what type of activity you want to do? Do you have the proper equipment, such as clothing and shoes, to get started? If you are going to a facility, is it in a convenient location or is it so far out of the way that the likelihood of going is small? Once you work out these details, see what happens. If you have all of the basics in place but still find yourself struggling, it's time to look at the meaning of exercise for you.

For most of your life, you've probably viewed exercise as a means to lose weight. As a result, exercise might feel like a punishment. It's a means of burning up the calories from the cake you weren't supposed to eat. It's a means of getting your body into the right shape, with the implication that your body is the wrong shape. As with a diet, the only indicator of the success of your exercise program is weight loss. If you don't become thinner, you've failed. All of these notions set you up to rebel. You're at risk of seeing exercise as an all-or-nothing proposition. As soon as you miss a time or two of your planned exercise, you feel you've blown it and stop completely—just as you are either on or off a diet. To improve the chances that you'll sustain whatever type of movement you choose, it's essential to let go of weight loss as your motivation.

Think about separating the notion of weight loss from exercise. This might take some time if they are connected at a deep level for you. Try reminding yourself frequently that the purpose of exercise isn't about weight loss. When you exercise, your body will respond according to your physiology. Some of you will become very fit and not lose an ounce of weight. That does not mean you're failing in any way. You're attaining all of the benefits that come from improving the fitness of your body, and you can feel proud that you're taking such good care of yourself. If you find that when you become physically active, your body changes in shape or size, remind yourself that this is a side effect and not the overriding goal. If you consider yourself successful because you lose weight through exercise, you're once again at risk of turning this caretaking behavior into some form of a diet.

Sometimes diet survivors discover that the obstacle getting in the way of exercise is that they believe that they will, in fact, lose weight. This may sound strange at first because the reason you have dieted in the past was for weight loss. Sometimes, on a deeper level, people have feelings or beliefs that contradict what they think they want. One diet survivor found that she was struggling to exercise because experience told her that she would lose weight once she started moving her body. However, her husband constantly hassled her about her size, and she realized that if she lost weight, she would feel like she was letting him win. She found her way out of this bind by realizing that it would give him just as much power if she did not exercise because he wanted her to as it would if she did exercise because he wanted her to. Ultimately, she had to decide what was caretaking for her, and act in accordance with her own needs.

It's a shame that the focus on weight loss is a major factor that gets in the way of people's ability to start and sustain physical activity. It's a shame that many doctors tell their larger patients to exercise with the expectation of weight loss, rather than recommending exercise to patients of all sizes as a means of improving physical and mental health. It's a shame that people stop exercising when they don't lose weight because they think it's not working.

You can make a different decision. Stop connecting weight loss and exercise and start moving your body. Focus on the positive aspects of integrating physical activity into your life.

ACTIVITY: Exercising Your Right to Self-Care

Imagine that exercise wouldn't result in weight loss for anyone, including you. List the reasons you might still want to exercise. Think about what benefits physical activity holds for you without putting weight loss into the mix.

1. _____
2. _____
3. _____
4. _____
5. _____

"Physical fitness is not only one of the most important keys to a healthy body, it is the basis of dynamic and creative intellectual activity."
—*John F. Kennedy*

LESSON #47

Learning to manage your feelings without food is a process that takes time. Allow yourself the space you need as you gently nudge yourself to be with your feelings.

How do you feel right now? Are you content or restless? Hopeful or scared? Angry or determined? Knowing how you feel gives you important information about yourself. It allows you to understand what is going on for you in a particular situation and can guide you in deciding how to live your life. Simply the act of identifying what you feel can lead to a greater sense of calmness.

In lesson #20, we explained that the day would come when you notice mouth hunger and decide that you can postpone eating. You are now in a stronger position to experience your feelings without turning to food, as the result of practicing attuned eating, acceptance, and self-care. Ask yourself often, "What would I think about or feel if I didn't eat right now?" The answer to this question will give you a window into your inner life.

Have you ever heard the phrase "sitting with your feelings"? From a psychological standpoint, this idea means that you're able to allow whatever you feel to be consciously on your mind, without trying to push the feeling away. Everyone experiences a wide range of feelings. Yet certain feelings such as anger or sadness can be hard to tolerate. There's no getting around the fact that everyone has difficult or painful feelings at various times in their life. Your task as a diet survivor who is trying to break the connection between food and feelings is to sit with these feelings without reaching for food.

It is important to practice identifying your feelings and tolerating them for as long as it takes to work your way through them. You cannot sidestep this process. Sitting with feelings means allowing yourself to go through the feeling in whatever way you need to at a particular time in your life.

Think about the idea of riding a wave. It moves along, reaches a peak, and then breaks as it rolls onto the shore. In a way, intense feelings go through a similar pattern. You may feel so mad at someone that you cannot believe you could ever forgive her. Yet, as the days pass, you realize your rage has diminished. You may find that your feelings naturally diminish as time passes, or you might use them to guide you in talking with that person about whatever is bothering you. In either case, the strength of your feelings will lessen. Keep reminding yourself that the intensity of your feelings will subside over time. Repeat to yourself, like a mantra, "this will pass."

Sometimes it's difficult to tolerate a particular feeling

because it seems unacceptable to you. You might feel frightened by the sexual attraction you feel toward your friend's boyfriend or guilty over the disappointment you feel in your child. It's important to remind yourself that a feeling is just a feeling. Just because you're aware of a particular emotion doesn't mean that you must act on it. You are in charge of deciding what you want to do about a feeling once you notice it exists. Give yourself permission to have your feelings without judgment. Let yourself sit with your feeling and then decide how you want to proceed.

Reaching for food is a way that you might have learned to manage uncomfortable feelings. As you increase your ability to feed yourself when you're physically hungry, you'll be in a stronger position to learn how to deal with your feelings without food. However, this skill won't happen magically or instantly. Rather, it requires you to understand the importance of allowing your full range of feelings and accepting whatever emotions arise. It also means letting yourself be with those feelings over a period of time so that you can figure out what to do. Sometimes identifying the feeling will be enough to help you feel calm; sometimes you'll need to figure out what action to take based on your feeling. There will be moments when you can tolerate your feelings and times when it just feels too hard, so you reach for food. Give yourself a gentle nudge in the direction of being with your feelings, and stay compassionate with yourself.

ACTIVITY: Riding the Wave

The next time you are sitting with a strong feeling, try to "ride the wave," using the following suggestions as guidelines:

- Label the feeling.
- Notice the feeling gathering momentum. With time, the feeling gathers force and feels as if it might drown you. Can you find a way to check in with yourself about the fears you may have in experiencing this emotion? Remind yourself that this is the height of the feeling wave and it will pass.
- The feeling will run its course to shore, and what was once large and foreboding dissipates in a sea of calmer waters. Check in with yourself and see what was useful as you rode out the crest of the wave. What might you want to try the next time you are faced with a strong feeling?
- Remind yourself that this is the nature of all feelings. Go with the flow!

"You can't stop the waves, but you can learn to surf."
—Jon Kabat Zinn

LESSON #48

As you develop the capacity to manage your feelings without food, you'll need to find other outlets. Develop strategies that will help you in times of discomfort.

Now that you're learning to identify your feelings and let them hang around for a while, you'll need to decide what to do next. Different people find that different techniques work for them. This is a time of experimentation for you.

As we've stated in previous lessons, sometimes it's enough just to identify a feeling. You may find yourself calmer and able to get through whatever emotion you're experiencing. Often, however, a feeling opens a door and needs further exploration. Initially, you may just want to mull over the feeling. Some diet survivors find it helpful to talk about the feeling out loud. By sharing your feelings, you can experience comfort as another person validates your experience or asks questions that help you explore your feelings. If you're usually the one people come to with problems, it can take some practice to switch roles. Remember that you're entitled to be the one in need at times. Make sure you find relationships in which you feel heard and understood. Sometimes people want to try to jump in and offer all kinds of suggestions to help you solve your problem. While their wish to help you is understandable, it's usually more useful when someone is able to use good listening skills and let you sort out your feelings without giving advice.

Other diet survivors find that keeping a journal is a wonderful way to explore their feelings. Allow yourself to write down whatever comes to mind. See if this way of keeping track of your thoughts and feelings provides a useful outlet as you work your way through emotions without turning to food.

There are other activities that are soothing. Taking a walk, reading a book, or watching a DVD may help you get through a time of discomfort. You can think of these types of activities as providing a calming function or serving as a distraction. There's nothing wrong with moving away from your feelings at times. After all, you cannot be expected to sit with your feelings constantly. By turning to these activities, you're not denying that you have a feeling. In the past, you may have participated in diet programs that also recommended these kinds of activities as ways to control your eating. We want to be clear about the difference. In those programs, the goal was to stop yourself from eating by doing something else. What we are suggesting is a different process in which you acknowledge what you're feeling and then make an active decision to calm yourself by engaging in a behavior that helps you in that moment. If you need to eat, you will. If you can get through the moment without food, you will. Both options are fine. In either case, you'll still try to understand what you're feeling.

You may also try to incorporate activities that enhance your overall well-being and contribute to your repertoire of coping skills. Meditation, the ancient art of relaxing your body and quieting your mind, increases your physical and emotional wellness. Humor is emotionally healing and has physical benefits as well. Developing a new hobby or following your passion for something gives you a way to express yourself and experience pleasure. All of these life-enhancing skills offer you ways to take care of yourself by strengthening you.

Diet survivors have no more or less emotional issues than normal eaters. However, if you find that when you stop using food to manage feelings you experience depression, anxiety, or other emotions that seem difficult to handle on your own, seek the help of a trained professional.

Think about what feels calming to you. How can you help yourself through a moment of discomfort without reaching for food? The fact that you have uncomfortable feelings is natural. The fact that you have a difficult time sitting with them is understandable. Your task is to find ways that let you be in touch with your feelings in a manner that is tolerable. Experiment with different techniques until you find solutions that feel caretaking.

ACTIVITY: Planning with Feeling

Make a list of things you could do when you're dealing with a strong emotion. Be specific. If you list talking with a friend, which friend are you referring to? If you want to watch a movie, which one is it? If you list journaling or painting, make sure you have the necessary supplies. Listing ways you might choose to work with strong emotions can help you feel supported and more directed in times of difficulty.

_____

_____

_____

_____

_____

"The emotions are sometimes so strong that I work without knowing it. The strokes come like speech."
—Vincent van Gogh

LESSON #49

Allow yourself some down time when you need it.
You don't have to eat when you're not hungry in
order to give yourself a break.

No matter how busy your life is, there are times when you need to stop what you're doing and take some time out for yourself. Many diet survivors give themselves a break by eating. This frequently occurs at the end of the day when you're trying to catch up on all of the tasks that need to be done in your home. You may believe that it's not okay to stop just because you need some down time. Instead, eating somehow gives you permission for taking that much needed break.

The problem is that there's always something else to be done. If you're at home at night or on the weekend, there's probably more laundry to wash, bills to pay, phone calls to return, and rooms to be straightened. If you wait until everything is done to give yourself a break, that time will never come. There's always more to do. Instead, think about giving yourself permission to take some time for yourself, even when all of your chores aren't completed yet.

Many people find that they eat when they are tired in order to try and stay awake for a longer period of time. However, as you become more in tune with your body, noticing that you are tired gives you important information. You are learning to respond to your internal cues by making good matches, and the best match for sleepiness is resting or going to bed rather than eating.

When you turn to food to give yourself a break, you're reaching for the wrong solution. It's okay that you need to stop what you're doing. You may be exhausted from your day and craving some quiet time. You do *not* have to eat in order to take a break.

What should you do instead of eating? You might read a magazine, watch television, or simply sit down and do nothing! You may find that a half-hour break energizes you so that you can complete a particular task. Or you may decide that you are done for the day. Only you can decide what's best for you.

You may protest that if you stop, important things will never get done. This, understandably, creates stress for you. Just as you've done with food, think about what would make the best "match" for you in a particular situation. Is it more satisfying to clean out the closet so that your home feels organized, or does it feel better to read another chapter of a book that you're really into? Figure out at a given moment what will feel the best to you. If you're reaching for food because you feel you should clean the closet but don't really want to, then you must stop and become more mindful of what's happening.

You can decide that cleaning the closet will feel worth it to you and keep going, or you can give yourself permission to stop and take the much-needed break. You don't need to eat when you're not hungry in order to make that choice. Of course, if cleaning the closet gave you an appetite, then by all means stop and feed yourself!

You may feel that at least you're doing something when you're eating. But reaching for food when you're not hungry is the wrong response to your need. Everyone needs to stop from time to time. Give yourself permission to take that time out for yourself. This might mean relaxing your standards about the neatness of your home. It might mean using the time you would spend eating to relax in a different manner. Stay aware of your own needs and stop judging yourself for not being able to do it all. The demands of today's lifestyles can feel overwhelming. You are only human. There is always more to do. Trust your body to know when it needs a break, and then take it!

ACTIVITY: Let's Break It Up

The following list includes examples of how food gets confused with giving yourself some time. Place a check next to the situations that apply to you, and then see if you can add other examples of your own.

1. Eating past fullness at dinner because you don't feel ready to move on to the evening tasks.

2. Eating in the afternoon because you're tired but feel you shouldn't nap.
3. Eating at night because you're tired but believe you can't go to bed yet.
4. Eating because you're bored with the activity you're engaged in.
5. _____
6. _____
7. _____

"Take rest; a field that has rested gives a bountiful crop."
—*Ovid*

LESSON #50

As you learn to become an attuned eater, you'll become more in tune with your whole self. Notice that you have needs in other areas of your life as well.

The basic act of feeding yourself can become a metaphor for meeting your needs in other areas of your life. As you check in with yourself to ask what you're hungry for, you're likely to check in with yourself about other needs as well. As you feel entitled to meet your needs by eating when you're hungry and choosing foods that are right for you, you're likely to feel more entitled to meet other types of needs. As you enjoy the satisfaction that comes from making a good match with your hunger, you're likely to feel satisfaction when you meet your other needs. As you see that there is enough food in the world to meet your hunger needs, you're more likely to feel that your other needs can be fulfilled as well.

So how does all of this wonderful stuff begin to happen? The key is to pay attention. You already know how to pay attention to physical hunger, and you're working toward identifying your feelings. The combination of these two skills will empower you to listen to other aspects of yourself.

What else do you hunger for? Do you need more friends in your life? Do you desire more activity or less?

Do you long to travel? Do you want to end a difficult relationship? Is your work life satisfying?

Here is how the experience of attuned eating translated to another area for one diet survivor. She was the primary caretaker of her elderly father, spending practically all of her free time taking care of him. She realized that she was exhausted and overwhelmed by these demands. As she felt more comfortable with the idea of listening to her hunger needs, she felt empowered to focus on her other needs. She held a meeting with her siblings and told them that she needed more support. She asked that they take on some of the responsibilities. To her surprise, they readily agreed. They hadn't been aware that she felt burdened by the caretaking needs of their father because she had always cheerfully offered to do them. Her capacity to create this change came from the combination of the positive reinforcement of meeting her needs through attuned eating along with her increased ability to identify her feelings.

Another diet survivor realized that she was pursuing the wrong career in graduate school. Her parents had expected her follow to in their footsteps and become a lawyer, and she had never questioned this. However, as she had success in making matches with food, she realized the difference between eating what she was supposed to versus eating what felt right to her. She then applied this skill to other areas of her life. When she was honest with herself, she acknowledged that she didn't feel she was in the right place at law school. The truth was that she was always drawn toward psychology, and that being a therapist felt like a much better fit with her personality. It was a difficult decision to leave law school because she didn't want to disappoint her parents. But she recognized that pursuing a degree in psychology was what would truly make her happy.

Another diet survivor felt that her needs were so huge that they could never be met. How could there possibly be enough love in the world to fill her longing to be loved? Who could possibly care enough for her to fill her emptiness? Yet, as she began to experience the fact that there was enough food available to fill her stomach, she was able to consider the possibility that her other needs were not endless. With the help of a counselor, she began to see that people could care for her. She was able to let herself take in the care from other people and to enjoy these connections.

How can the process of normalizing your eating lead to such dramatic changes? The act of feeding yourself in accordance with your needs is a powerful tool. Once you experience how much better you feel when you listen to your needs, there is no turning back. Listening to your needs is an act of self-care that will increase the quality of your life.

Of course, just because you recognize your needs doesn't mean that you'll be able to meet them perfectly each and every time. As with food, sometimes you'll need to decide what makes a good enough match. Sometimes your needs will compete, such as when it would feel like a good match to go out to lunch with a friend at the same time that it would feel like a good match to use that time to accomplish a task at work. However, overall you'll find that you can live your life in accordance with your needs most of the time, and your life will become more satisfying.

Use the metaphors of attuned eating as much as possible. Ask yourself what you "hunger" for. Think about what would make a good "match." Ask yourself if an experience or interaction felt "satisfying." This approach will help you learn more about who you are and what you need.

ACTIVITY: Attuned Living

Fill in the blanks in the following paragraph to identify how you can translate the principles of attuned eating into the practice of attuned living.

One thing that I know I am *hungry* for is

_____

I think a good *match* to this hunger/need is

_____

because

_____

_____

_____

I trust that I can meet this need and be *satisfied* because I know that

_____

_____

_____

"Go confidently in the direction of your dreams.
Live the life you have imagined."
—Henry David Thoreau

LESSON #51

It is never selfish to listen to your own needs. When you take care of yourself you're in a stronger position to take care of others.

Think about what it means to take care of your own needs. Does the word *selfish* come to mind? If so, you're not alone. Many diet survivors believe that they should think about the needs of other people, rather than their own.

There are all sorts of reasons for this belief. Your parents may have taught you that it's selfish to think about yourself. You may believe, consciously or unconsciously, that the way to get attention or love from other people is to do things for them. Whatever the cause for this belief, the result is that you actively disregard your own needs.

When you count on other people to take care of your needs, you put yourself in a precarious position. First, nobody knows better than you what you need at a particular moment. Second, there are some things that only you can do for yourself. No one else can relax for you, exercise for you, identify what you need to eat, or fulfill your dreams. If you wait for someone else to fill your needs, there's a good chance they will go unmet.

Furthermore, if you are someone who constantly takes care of other people—without taking care of yourself—

there's a good chance that you feel resentful. This does-n't mean you're selfish! Feeling resentful or burdened is a natural response to the depletion that comes from using up so much energy for other people without replenishing yourself. The best thing that you can do for yourself and for the important people in your life is to make sure that your needs are met.

Taking the time to care for yourself is never a selfish act. You deserve to feel good in life and to preserve the boundaries between yourself and others so that your needs are met. Think of this task as a balancing act. No one can meet every single need at the moment it arises. If you're at work and have an urge to have a conversation with your best friend, it will probably have to wait. But you can call her after you go home. Sometimes you have to make difficult choices. If you would prefer to go to a movie with your significant other but your sick aunt needs someone to take her to the hospital, what will you do? You may value helping your aunt enough that you cancel your plans. But what if she needs you for some-thing minor instead? Is it still okay with you to cancel your plans? At what point do you ask that another rela-tive help if her demands become more constant? Or, if there is no one else, at what point do you explain to her that she must plan ahead so that you can arrange your schedule in a way that works for both of you? You can care very much about someone, but still be unable to do things all of the time. This is not selfish. This is reality!

Boundaries are extremely important. They are the line between what is okay for you and what is not. You are in charge of where those boundaries are. Boundaries protect you from becoming overwhelmed and burdened by the needs of others. When you don't set boundaries for yourself, you're at risk of turning to food to manage these feelings.

According to the dictionary, being selfish means caring *only* for oneself. If, in fact, you thought only about yourself all of the time, that would be selfish. However, the definition does not say that you should *never* think about yourself. In healthy relationships, needs of both people get met. In the best of all worlds, there is a sense of reciprocity in relationships. You do for others and they do for you. However, none of us can get *all* of our needs met through other people, no matter how good those relationships might be. We all have the responsibility of identifying and meeting our own needs.

When you take care of yourself, you will feel better. You might find yourself more energetic, calmer, and more optimistic. And then, when the time is right, you'll be better able to help another person. Remember, taking actions to make yourself happier isn't selfish. In fact, when you do feel more grounded, doing things for others can feel quite wonderful!

ACTIVITY: Don't put me on hold!

Before every plane takes off, the flight attendant goes over the safety features of the aircraft. As the crew demonstrates the oxygen mask falling in the event of an emergency, they explain that adults should use the mask themselves first, before assisting children. This is an important lesson not only when you fly in a plane, but when you fly through life as well. Take a moment to make a list of times this past week when you put your own needs on hold.

_____

_____

_____

From that list, pick one unmet need and answer the following questions:

Where were you and what you were you doing?

_____

_____

_____

What need did you put on hold?

_____

_____

_____

Why did you put that need on hold?

_____

_____

_____

How did you feel when your need wasn't met?

_____

_____

_____

Is this a need you often put on hold?

_____

_____

_____

What were the consequences of putting that need on hold?

_____

_____

_____

> *"If I am not for myself,*
> *Who will be for me?*
> *If I am only for myself,*
> *What am I?*
> *If not now,*
> *When?"*
> *—Rabbi Hillel*

LESSON #52

Let go of perfectionist thinking and learn to determine what's good enough. Rarely are things black or white.

Many diet survivors set very high standards for themselves. Whether it's in their work life or home life, they want everything to be perfect. If this describes you, then you know how important if feels to maintain these standards. Anything less means failure.

Perfectionist thinking can manifest itself in different ways. From the outside, it may look to others like you've got it all. Your home is beautiful. You're successful at school, in your job, or in your volunteer work. You always appear put together when you go out. Everything seems great.

Perfectionist thinking may be evident in how you approach things. There's a feeling that you have to get it right the first time. If you don't, you're a failure. You see the world in all-or-nothing terms. There is no room for a learning curve. Either you've got it or you don't. You assign judgment to yourself so that you're good when you get it right and bad when you don't.

If you're a perfectionist, the problem for you is that you experience a tremendous amount of anxiety. The nature of being perfect means one misstep and you're a failure. That's a heavy burden to carry. For whatever purpose your perfectionism serves, you're scared to let it go. You hang onto it despite the fact that the anxiety it creates might lead to soothing yourself with food.

There is an alternative to perfectionist thinking: reevaluating your standards and deciding what is good enough. How clean does your house have to be to feel acceptable, without completely draining you? How important is it really to stay an extra hour at work in order to return every phone call when it's the first beautiful day of summer and you crave a walk? So what if you haven't mastered the song you're working on in time for your next piano lesson? The world will not come to an end.

Being a diet survivor *and* a perfectionist thinker creates challenges. Diets have clear rules to follow. You feel like a success when you follow the rules—and you will follow them perfectly at first—only to feel like a complete failure when you stray from the plan. Diets promote the all-or-nothing concepts of good and bad, on and off. As you work through the lessons in this book, you're engaged in a very different sort of process that requires you to suspend your perfectionism. There are still guidelines to follow as you identify hunger, make matches, notice fullness, end judgments, and learn how to deal with feelings. However, there's no expectation that you'll master these tasks perfectly. Instead, there's the acknowledgment that implementing these goals take practice over a period of time. Rather than thinking in terms of success and failure, work toward letting go of this black-or-white thinking, and see what it's like to live in the gray area.

All people have strengths and weaknesses. That is nothing to be ashamed of. Celebrate your strengths and use them to the best of your ability. Evaluate your weaknesses. Decide what you can change and what is just a part of who you are. None of us can get everything right all of the time.

Examine the words you use to talk to yourself about your standards. If you frequently use phrases such as "I should" or "I must," then you need to gently challenge yourself. Don't expect to let go of these beliefs right away—that would be the perfectionist part of you placing unrealistic demands on yourself yet again! Instead, as you catch yourself thinking in perfectionist ways, gently remind yourself that you're trying to move away from these patterns. Think about what is good enough. Think about where the middle lies between perfection and failure. Think about process rather than outcome. Stop thinking in black-and-white terms. Go gray!

ACTIVITY: In a Perfect World, I Wouldn't Have to Be So Perfect

Gently try to challenge perfectionist thinking by exploring how you've been speaking to yourself and how those words direct your actions.

Pick a category from the following list:

- Family
- Friends
- Work
- Home

Can you identify perfectionist thinking in that area? The words commonly used in perfectionist standards include "I must" and "I should."

Write down your perfectionist standard.

_____

_____

_____

Write down why you believe this is true.

_____

_____

_____

Challenge your reasoning about this belief.

_____

_____

_____

Write a sentence that reflects a more middle ground.

_____

_____

_____

Remember, you don't have to be purfekt!

"They tell you that nobody is perfect. Then they tell you that practice makes perfect. I wish they'd make up their minds."
—Winston Churchill

LESSON #53

Make sure that you own your own feelings.
Remind yourself that you're not responsible for the
feelings of others.

Consider the phrase "owning your feelings." This means acknowledging your feelings to yourself and others, and taking responsibility for the way you feel. Diet survivors frequently prefer to avoid conflict. If this applies to you, then there are times that you don't acknowledge your feelings because you fear how it will affect your relationships.

One diet survivor described a situation with her husband. He repeatedly asked her to pick up his dry cleaning, and she repeatedly forgot. She didn't want to annoy him deliberately, yet there was a reason she forgot. She felt resentful that he didn't value her time and did not seem to truly get just what went into running a household and taking care of young children. Forgetting to do an errand for him was her way of expressing that feeling. She needed to own her feelings and honestly tell her husband that she felt unappreciated.

The biggest reason that diet survivors have difficulty owning their feelings is that they're afraid of the reaction of another person. One diet survivor found herself in a financial bind because she believed she was responsible for the feelings of others. During the fall, she agreed to go on vacation with her sister the following summer. However, due to layoffs at her company, she was unexpectedly unemployed and no longer had the income to spend on a luxury trip. She didn't want to upset her sister and never let on that this vacation would put her into debt. If she had cancelled the trip, her sister probably would've felt disappointed. That's okay. She's entitled to feel disappointed. However, this diet survivor was still entitled to cancel her trip. Sometimes needs conflict, and there's no getting around that. In healthy relationships, people stay respectful of each other and can tolerate the difficult feelings that will naturally arise at times. You cannot control how other people feel. You can only take responsibility for the way you feel and hope that others will do the same.

Here's another example. Your friend asks you where you would like to go for dinner. You tell her that you don't care, even though you would like Italian food. She chooses a Greek restaurant, which does not meet your needs. What were you afraid of? If you told her you wanted Italian food, and she did not, she was free to let you know. Then the two of you could have found some sort of compromise. If she went along with your suggestion of an Italian restaurant just because she was uncomfortable saying no, that's her issue. You cannot spend your life second-guessing the needs of others. Each of you must take responsibility for your own feelings.

Furthermore, when you opted out by saying you don't care where you eat, your friend might have felt frustrated that she had to make the decision for both of you. It's actually easier in the long run if you say what you want, she says what she wants, and then both of you take it from there. When people have to guess what others want, decisions become convoluted, and no one's needs may be met. It might turn out that you were on the same page already, but if not, the nature of good relationships is that you can work things out.

What will happen if you start to own your own feelings and someone gets angry with you? That's probably exactly what you've been trying to avoid. Sometimes when you start to make changes, it means that the people around you have to make adjustments too. Some will be able to do that, but some may not. If they cannot, the relationship may be in jeopardy. We do not say this lightly, and we know that this can feel scary to you. However, if you are in relationships where people cannot listen to you or respect your needs, your relationship is already in trouble. You will need to evaluate which relationships support your well-being and decide how to take care of yourself if you find yourself in relationships that require you to sacrifice your well-being.

Take responsibility for your feelings. Let people know in a respectful way whatever you need, want, or feel. And let them react in the way that they need to as well. As difficult as it might be, when people are direct with each other, it creates opportunities for growth.

ACTIVITY: What I Feel Is...

These steps will help you practice owning your feelings.

Step One:

Determine what you are feeling. Sometimes we want to hide our feelings, even from ourselves. Pay close attention to your feelings in different situations.

Step Two:

Acknowledge those feelings in relationships. As you become more comfortable naming your feelings to yourself, practice putting them out there. It might be voicing your movie preference with a friend or sharing with your partner your wish to spend more time together.

Step Three:

Listen to and hear the feelings expressed by the other person; you're both entitled to own your feelings and express yourselves.

Step Four:

Practice sitting with a level of discomfort. Owning and voicing your feelings paves the way for healthier relationships. Tension resulting from honest expression from your feelings and those of others creates an opportunity to use that tension to move the relationship forward in new ways.

"Be who you are and say what you feel because those who mind don't matter and those who matter don't mind."
—Dr. Seuss

LESSON #54

Learn to become comfortable with the idea of having
two sets of different feelings at the same time.

You are in the process of getting better at noticing your feelings. By doing so, you can make better decisions about how you want to live your life. However, one of the biggest reasons that diet survivors turn to food to numb or distract themselves from their emotions is because certain thoughts or feelings seem unacceptable. This may happen at times because your feelings are at odds with each other. Here's how it works.

Let's say you have just decided to take a job in a new city. You are excited about the position and feel that this is a good step for you. At the same time, however, you feel an incredible sense of loss. You will be moving away from your close friends to an unfamiliar community. You feel sad and scared. You question whether you have made a wise decision. So which is valid? Your excitement or your sadness? The thrill of a new challenge or the fear of leaving the familiar?

You can make room for both kinds of feelings. It makes as much sense that you are scared and sad as that you are excited. They are just two different sets of feelings, and they *can* coexist. Some people may try to talk you out of your sad feelings by telling you to stay positive, that it will all work out. Allowing yourself to feel your sadness in no way means that you are not a positive person. You can look forward to the challenge of the move and still feel sad. And probably things will work out fine. However, it would be better if your friend could let you acknowledge both; it will be hard to leave *and* it is exciting. Notice that we did not say, "It will be hard to leave, *but* it is exciting." In this sentence, the word "but" implies that there isn't room for both feelings at the same time. There is! You are sad *and* excited. You do not have to make either feeling go away.

Now consider another situation that is complicated on an emotional level. You are angry with your mother because you have realized that she was never able to truly understand your needs as a child. She always seemed more concerned about how certain events or situations affected her, and therefore never understood your experience. After a while, you gave up trying to get her to listen and kept your feelings to yourself. Now, when you acknowledge your anger, you feel disloyal toward your mother. After all, she is a good person and you know she loves you—so you try to make your anger go away.

Here is the dilemma. If you allow yourself to experience only your positive feelings toward your mother, you must deny your own authentic experience. You must pretend that your anger does not exist or minimize its importance. Any time that feelings of anger or disappointment threaten to surface, they will feel unacceptable to you. Reaching for food when you are not hungry is one way that you try to keep these feelings at bay. If, on the other hand, you allow yourself to feel disappointment or rage, while believing that these strong emotions negate your positive feelings toward your mother, it will be very scary. When these intense feelings surface, you will again be at risk of trying to deal with them by turning to food.

The solution to this problem is to allow yourself to acknowledge *both* sets of your very real feelings. Your mother did the best she could to take good care of you in many ways *and,* at the same time, she let you down in many ways. One realization does not negate the other.

Human beings lead intricate emotional lives. When you have two sets of feelings that seem contradictory, it does not mean you cannot make up your mind. Rather, you have the capacity to feel different emotions about the same person or situation at the same time. If you can accept that this is both possible and natural, you will not need to try to make one set of feelings go away in order to justify the other. Instead, you can become comfortable with the notion that you are a complex person with many thoughts, feelings, and ideas.

ACTIVITY: Yin and Yang

The yin-yang symbol is an ancient Chinese expression of how the world works. The outer circle symbolizes everything, while the shapes within the circle represent the interaction of two energies: yin (black) and yang (white). The yin and yang embody the opposite principles of the universe: yin represents the principle of femaleness, and yang represents maleness. By placing a small circle of white in the black area and a small circle of black in the white area, the symbol further represents the notion that nothing in life—including emotion—is all black or all white. The two energies reflect the continual movement of forces and the cyclical nature of phenomena.

Can you think of an occasion when you were aware of experiencing different feelings at the same time? Take time to really think about that experience, and allow the different feelings to surface. Write down both emotional states on the line below.

_____

Allow yourself to take in both the complexity and simplicity of experiencing different feelings at the same time. Feelings are both fluid and interactive.

> *"It is very hard to say the exact truth, even about your own immediate feelings—much harder than to say something fine about them which is not the exact truth."*
> —George Eliot

LESSON #55

Reaching for food when you're not hungry can become an opportunity to learn something important about yourself. Welcome these moments.

As you normalize your eating and end the use of food to manage feelings, wonderful things happen! You no longer spend a lot of mental energy thinking or worrying about food. You deal with your problems head-on. You experience satisfaction and pleasure when it comes to eating.

Does this mean that you will never eat again when you're not hungry? Absolutely not! Normal eaters eat in response to physical cues *most* of the time; everyone occasionally eats for reasons other than physical hunger. If this happens to you from time to time because something at a party looks too good to pass up or because you eat a bit more of a food than you need, don't worry. Stay aware of how your body feels and return to responding to internal cues as soon as possible.

If you find that you're eating out of physiological hunger most of the time and then experience a surge in overeating that is perplexing to you, think of it as an opportunity to learn something important about yourself. If you're a diet survivor who has used food in the past to manage uncomfortable feelings, you have a vulnerability to return to food for calming. While you're developing the capacity to handle your feelings without food most of the time, there might be moments when you return to food—or thoughts of food—for comfort. Don't fret. Instead, welcome these moments as opportunities to become aware that something is going on inside of yourself. Think of this reach for food as a window into your emotional life.

One diet survivor noticed that after months of eating in an attuned manner, she found herself having donuts and cake at work, even though she really did not want them. She checked to make sure that all of the basics of this approach were in place; she was well-stocked at home and work, she was not judging foods as "good" or "bad," and she was listening to her body regarding hunger, matching, and fullness. She then began to ask herself what could possibly be bothering her. She traced back her last experience of eating the sweets when she was not hungry and thought about what had been on her mind at the time. She realized that she was feeling upset with her husband for missing a family reunion because of a work crisis. She had told him that she understood his need to choose work over the family gathering. However, deep down she felt disappointed and questioned whether he could have figured out a way to manage his work around this event. She even wondered if he would have found a way if it were his family that was having the reunion. She had been trying to push back these feelings, and her mouth hunger was her mind's way of letting her know that she needed to attend to them. She decided to speak directly to her husband about her feelings, and expressing them was a relief to her, even though it did not change what had already happened. Identifying her feelings allowed her to resume her attuned eating.

Another diet survivor had normalized her eating and done a lot of work on managing her feelings so that she could tolerate the loneliness she experienced in the evening. It surprised her when she noticed an increase in mouth hunger at night. Rather than yelling at herself for overeating, she became curious. She asked herself what she would be thinking about or feeling if she did not reach for food at that moment. To her surprise, it had nothing to do with the lonely feelings that were often present in the evening. Instead, she realized she felt dread about going to work in the mornings. Recently, her boss with whom she had a wonderful relationship had left her job, and the new boss was turning out to be difficult. Although she realized that she was concerned about this new boss, she hadn't been aware of just how anxious she was. She loved her job, but felt that there was a real possibility that she couldn't stay under the direction of this new person. Although there was nothing to do for the moment, it was important for her to acknowledge her fear and to begin brainstorming alternatives should things not work out.

In both of these examples, mouth hunger was the signal that an emotional issue needed to be addressed. You have a history of turning to food when you're in emotional trouble. It was good that you tried to help yourself during that time, but it was the wrong solution to your difficulties. You needed to face your feelings and problems directly. If you've accomplished this task most of the time, you've made a tremendous positive change in your life. Yet once in awhile you might unconsciously rely on this old behavior to alert you that something is up. Don't ignore this reach for food. Instead, welcome the opportunity to check in with yourself and see what important feelings are waiting to be discovered.

ACTIVITY: Looking for Signs

Your behavior has meaning. Come to know the signs that inform you that something is up. Use the road map below to help you determine the meaning of this detour from your usual pattern of attuned eating.

Stop! What changes have you noticed in your eating? (Are you restricting? Are you overeating?)

Caution! What emotions might be contributing to the change in your eating?

Yield! Remain gentle with yourself as you explore your feelings. What might your nurturing voice say?

Go! Keep moving in your process. The more you can stay open and curious, the more you can learn about yourself!

"Buddha left a road map, Jesus left a road map, Krishna left a road map, Rand McNally left a road map. But you still have to travel the road yourself."
—*Stephen Levine*

LESSON #56

Connect with the spiritual part of yourself.

Think about whether you give adequate attention to your spiritual self, the part of your being that feels connected to something bigger in the universe. There are many ways to experience your spirituality, such as through a connection with nature or belief in a higher power.

People who are spiritual may or may not believe in God. Spirituality gives you a sense of purpose in your life. It can determine your values and ethics and help you direct your energy into the world. It can provide you with important rituals and means to honor yourself and others. Views of life and death are intertwined with your spiritual self.

What helps *you* to feel a sense of awesomeness about the universe and your place in it? Is it gazing at the beauty of nature? Is it participating in an organized religious service? Is it yoga or meditation? As lives get busier and the cultural focus on material gain increases, it's easy to lose touch with your spiritual side. The constant noise that results from technology through the use of headphones, cell phones, and computers means that it is frequently easier to check out than to check in. Take time to ask yourself if you have enough quietness in your life to experience that deep awareness of yourself in relation to the world.

For many diet survivors, spirituality plays a role in managing feelings. You might find a comfort in your spiritual beliefs that helps you get through tough times without food. You might find ways in which your spiritual practices provide a soothing function that lets you be with whatever is on your mind without turning to food. Greater connection to yourself leads to better self-care.

Spirituality is a guiding force based on the principles of mindfulness, compassion, and wisdom. These ideas are paramount also to the way you feed yourself as you stay mindful of your hunger, compassionate with yourself, and in touch with the wisdom of your body to guide your eating. Staying in touch with your spirituality helps you to feed your soul.

ACTIVITY: Namaste

Namaste (pronounced *nama-stay*) is a Sanskrit greeting meaning "hello" and "good-bye." Namaste can be translated as: The divine in me recognizes and honors the divine in you. Typically, namaste is said while putting the hands together in a prayer position in front of the heart.

During the next week, take time to connect with your spiritual self. Where can you honor your own spirit, and in doing so, honor the spirit of others? Where do you feel connected on a deep level? Where do you feel a part of a wholeness that moves beyond words?

Take time and go there. It might be a walk at dawn or a service at a church, synagogue, or mosque. It might be sitting in meditation, prayer, or breathing in the scent of the rain. It might be reading from a spiritual work that moves you or writing your own words. Let yourself dance in the movement of life and in your sacred part of the whole.

"People travel to wonder at the height of mountains, at the huge waves of the sea, at the long courses of rivers, at the vast compass of the ocean, at the circular motion of the stars; and they pass by themselves without wondering."
—St. Augustine

LESSON #57

Avoid diet conversations: They are boring, encourage competition among women, and keep you from knowing your true nature and spirit.

As a diet survivor, you well know the endless conversations shared among friends, family, and colleagues regarding the topic of diets, weight, and body size. In this culture, women are encouraged to be concerned with the minutiae of their bodies and to bond together in sisterhood over body hatred. It is no coincidence that the current cultural ideal of extreme slenderness became popularized in the 1960s, during the time that women were enjoying economic and political gains. As women began taking up more space in the world, a backlash occurred where, implicitly, women were told to take up less space by being concerned with making their bodies smaller.

What is the cost for creative, intelligent, and passionate women to direct these qualities into the relentless pursuit of thinness? How many conversations focus on weight at the expense of sharing important ideas and insights about yourself, each other, and the world?

Think about realistic ways to move away from diet conversations. Refuse to take part in the endless diet talk that acts as an obstacle to the rewarding conversations that are a part of living a rich life. This means committing yourself to refrain from initiating diet conversations and exploring ways to redirect diet conversations initiated by others.

ACTIVITY: An Invitation

You're invited to a party to celebrate your spirit and share in conversation with other wonderful women!

What to bring: Your hopes, fears, and dreams.

What to leave behind: Diet talk, weight concerns, and negative thoughts about yourself.

As you prepare to attend this party, think about the following:

- What do you value in this life?
- What do you dream about, and what sustains you?
- What do you cherish?
- What are the unique gifts you offer to yourself and others?
- How do you want to spend your days? Your weeks? Your months? Your years?

When you no longer spend precious time dieting or talking about dieting, you allow yourself to connect with yourself and others in a deep and meaningful way.

"How we spend our days is, of course, how we spend our lives."
—Annie Dillard

LESSON #58

Build a support system for yourself. It's never easy to go against cultural expectations.

As a diet survivor, you're in the process of actively rejecting dieting as a method to improve your life. This decision takes courage. At times you might want to share and celebrate your new insights and accomplishments, and at other times you might need guidance or encouragement as you integrate attuned eating and acceptance into your life.

You are actively changing your relationship with food and integrating a whole new set of attitudes and beliefs. It will take time for other people to understand and accept your new approach. Finding others who can reinforce the soundness of your choice not to diet will go a long way in strengthening your resolve.

In the past, you might have tackled eating and weight issues in a formal setting, such as through a diet or weight management program. Usually, these sessions include groups where participants share their progress and experiences. Although it's validating to hear about the struggles of others who share similar problems, the focus of these groups is on the necessity of weight loss and controlled eating. People generally feel successful when pounds are shed and like a diet failure when weight isn't lost or the pounds return.

Coming together with a group of people who have actively decided to quit dieting and instead practice attuned eating and self-acceptance creates a safe and nurturing environment to explore important issues. This type of group, which can be led by a professional or set up more informally, focuses on moving in the direction of attuned eating and building a positive body image. The effects of these groups are powerful as members share feelings, thoughts, and experiences that influence their process in normalizing eating. Connection between members is based on supporting, validating, and helping each other to make peace with food and their bodies. As members share the details of their eating experiences and their negative body thoughts, feelings of shame—which are so often part of the dieter's psyche—are shifted to feelings of empowerment.

You've made a wise choice to stop dieting. But your resolve will be challenged at times. On days that you feel stronger, your internal voice will remind you that you've been there, done that. You'll remember that if diets really worked, people wouldn't need to return to them time after time. On days that you feel weaker, you may wonder if you should give dieting one last try. These feelings are normal and to be expected. However, it's in these moments that you must actively seek support for yourself to help you continue on the important journey you've begun.

ACTIVITY: Bring in the Reinforcements

There are numerous resources that offer a non-diet perspective. Choose one resource from any of the following categories and use the information you learn to reinforce your commitment to end dieting.

Books:

Beyond a Shadow of a Diet by Judith Matz and Ellen Frankel

Breaking Free from Compulsive Eating by Geneen Roth

Intuitive Eating by Evelyn Tribole and Elyse Resch

It's Not about Food by Carol Emery Normandi and Laurelee Roark

Moving Away from Diets by Karen Kratina, Nancy King, and Dayle Hayes

Overcoming Overeating by Jane Hirschmann and Carol Munter

Rules of Normal Eating by Karen Koenig

When Women Stop Hating Their Bodies by Jane Hirschmann and Carol Munter

Websites:

Beyond a Shadow of a Diet

www.beyondashadowofadiet.com

Healthy Weight Network

www.healthyweightnetwork.com
International No-Diet Day
www.eskimo.com/~largesse/INDD
National Center for Overcoming Overeating
www.overcomingovereating.com

> *"I can't understand why people are frightened by new ideas.*
> *I'm frightened by the old ones."*
> —*John Cage*

LESSON #59

Redefine your view of success. Work toward letting go of any shame that lingers.

We began this book by defining a *diet survivor* as any person who has been on more than one diet, lost and regained the weight, and is in the process of becoming aware that the failure isn't her fault. To the extent that you have integrated the information in these lessons into your psyche, your feelings of shame have decreased. No longer do you believe that you are lazy, bad, weak, or helpless. You understand that these feelings were created by the faulty messages you received from others about dieting and weight loss and reinforced by the advertising and dieting industries, which profited from your shame.

As you reject the cultural messages that suggest anyone can and should get thinner, you empower yourself. You open up the possibilities of redirecting your energies to other types of success that are within your reach. You *can* eat normally. You *can* take good care of your body. And you *can* take good care of yourself. There is no single definition or measure of success. Just as you are unique, your successes are unique.

What should you do about any shame that lingers? Given how deep that feeling might run, it will take some time to let it go fully. Make sure that you are not using your body to speak to yourself about shame generated by other experiences in your life. Stay gentle, and keep working to strengthen yourself by returning to these lessons as often as you need.

We must also stay hopeful of changing cultural messages about dieting and weight. If you started to get different messages from professionals, media, researchers, and others that eating according to your physical hunger is important and that you can work toward health at any size, your shame would decrease even more. That change may not be too far away, as more and more research validates these concepts.

Celebrate the successes that you've had with your accomplishments so far. Understanding that your failure with diets wasn't your fault was a huge hurdle to overcome. In doing so, you've opened yourself up to the possibilities of living a life that cannot be measured on a scale. You've increased your wellness and decreased your shame. No matter how far you've come—or how far you still have to go—your success is in the fact that you're making the journey.

ACTIVITY: To: Me, From: Me

Congratulations! It's time to celebrate your journey as a diet survivor. You've bought many cards for family and friends; now it's time to make one for yourself. What would you like to express to yourself about your accomplishments in the areas of eating, acceptance, and self-care? You might want to put your favorite quote or poem on the card, or write yourself a special message. Perhaps you want to include a picture that conveys your love of mountains, horses, or flowers. This is your chance to create a greeting card for yourself about the meaning of success, and the ways in which you are living a full life. Be creative! Get out all that fun stuff, like construction paper, scissors, glue, and markers, or create a card on the computer. Don't worry about being artistic—just have fun.

After you are finished, consider placing the card somewhere special where you can look to it as an affirmation of your worth that reflects your new definition of success.

"Success is liking yourself, liking what you do, and liking how you do it."
—Maya Angelou

LESSON #60

Consider sharing your experiences as a diet survivor.
You're in a position to empower others.

As you've worked toward normalizing your eating, accepting yourself, and engaging in self-care, you've accumulated numerous experiences. Do any of them stand out to you? Was there a moment when something felt particularly exciting or moving? If so, consider sharing your experience.

As people make changes, one of the most helpful tools is to hear about others in a similar situation who were able to overcome obstacles and achieve success. Your story is important. Other people who have not yet stopped dieting or who are in the early stages of doing so can benefit from what you have to say. Perhaps there was a moment when the connection between eating and hunger clicked for you. Or maybe there was a time when you discovered that allowing yourself to bring in previously "forbidden" foods led to an experience where you could enjoy that food when hungry, without overeating. Was there a moment of self-acceptance that felt truly profound? Are you able to live your life differently because of the peace you've made with food and yourself? Whatever feelings and experiences this process has generated for you, they have the potential to transform the life of someone else. Think of how you can share your experiences in a manner that feels comfortable. When you do so, you'll empower others by offering your courage and inspiration.

ACTIVITY: The Diet Survivor's Challenge

The activities in this book so far have been for your own personal use. Now, consider writing about your experiences for others to see. To learn more about this project, go to our website at www.dietsurvivors.com. Your voice is important, and we want to hear from you!

"Live your life from your heart. Share from your heart. And your story will touch and heal people's souls."
—Melody Beattie

Final Thoughts

"Nobody has ever measured, not even poets, how much the heart can hold."
—Zelda Fitzgerald

Hereyou are at the end of our book, but not at the end of your journey. We want to honor you for your courage in challenging the cultural norms and your wisdom in following a different path.

This book is about nourishing yourself. When you free yourself from dieting, your relationship with food changes in ways that you may never have imagined. You can eat for satiation and pleasure without anxiety. You are able to listen to your body and trust what it tells you. You are able to eat with gusto!

When you free yourself from the pressures of thinness, you experience your body in a new way. You can develop an attitude of acceptance toward yourself and others and move through the world with confidence. You are able to strengthen yourself.

When you free yourself from the obsession with food and weight, you free up a tremendous amount of energy for other pursuits. You are able to take in the beauty of the world that surrounds you in nature, develop relationships that nurture your soul, and invest yourself in work and activities that bring true satisfaction. You are able to live a full life.

So, dear reader, you get to take it from here. Celebrate your decision not to diet. Live well, eat well, and be well. Remember that we are with you in spirit on your journey. Take us with you and turn to these pages as often as you need. Always remember to keep your heart full and your stomach satisfied.

About the Authors

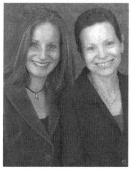

photo © Mark Chamberlain

Judith Matz, LCSW, and Ellen Frankel, LCSW, are clinical social workers and sisters who grew up in the Chicago area. In 2004 they published *Beyond a Shadow of a Diet: The Therapist's Guide to Treating Compulsive Eating.*

Judith is the director of the Chicago Center for Overcoming Overeating, Inc., an organization dedicated to ending the preoccupation with food and weight. She has worked in the area of eating problems since 1986 and is a frequent speaker at workshops and conferences on the topics of compulsive eating and body image. She has a private practice in Skokie, Illinois.

Ellen has worked in the field of eating disorders since 1987 in both outpatient and residential settings. Her book *Beyond Measure: A Memoir about Short Stature and Inner Growth* will be published in 2006. In addition to writing full time, she speaks at conferences and serves as a consultant. Ellen lives in Marblehead, Massachusetts.

You can visit their website at www.dietsurvivors.com.